Extended-Matching Questions for Finals

Commissioning Editor: Laurence Hunter
Development Editor: Ailsa Laing
Project Manager: Nancy Arnott
Designer: Erik Bigland

Extended-Matching Questions for Finals

John C. Alcolado
DM BM(Hons) PGCMedEd FRCP
Reader in Medicine
University of Cardiff School of Medicine
Cardiff, UK

M. Afzal Mir
DCH FRCP
Former Senior Lecturer & Consultant Physician
University Hospital of Wales
Cardiff, UK

SECOND EDITION

CHURCHILL LIVINGSTONE

ELSEVIER

EDINBURGH LONDON NEW YORK OXFORD PHILADELPHIA ST LOUIS SYDNEY TORONTO 2007

CHURCHILL
LIVINGSTONE
ELSEVIER

© Harcourt Publishers Limited 2002
© Elsevier Limited 2007

First edition 2002
Second edition 2007

ISBN   978-0-443-10376-6
ISBN   0-443-10376-3

British Library Cataloguing in Publication Data
A catalogue record for this book is available from the British Library

Library of Congress Cataloging in Publication Data
A catalog record for this book is available from the Library of Congress

Notice
Knowledge and best practice in this field are constantly changing. As new
research and experience broaden our knowledge, changes in practice,
treatment and drug therapy may become necessary or appropriate. Readers
are advised to check the most current information provided (i) on procedures
featured or (ii) by the manufacturer of each product to be administered, to
verify the recommended dose or formula, the method and duration of
administration, and contraindications. It is the responsibility of the
practitioner, relying on their own experience and knowledge of the patient,
to make diagnoses, to determine dosages and the best treatment for each
individual patient, and to take all appropriate safety precautions. To the
fullest extent of the law, neither the Publisher nor the Editors assume any
liability for any injury and/or damage to persons or property arising out of
or related to any use of the material contained in this book.

The Publisher

your source for books,
journals and multimedia
in the health sciences

www.elsevierhealth.com

The
publisher's
policy is to use
**paper manufactured
from sustainable forests**

Printed in China

Preface to the Second Edition

Since we wrote the first edition of *Extended-Matching Questions for Finals*, the extended-matching question (EMQ) format has been widely adopted in both undergraduate and postgraduate examinations in the UK and abroad.

We are aware that our book has been used in several ways by students, other than just as a source of sample questions. First, it is possible to use the lists in each theme as a quick revision aid of the common causes, symptoms, signs or diagnoses that are relevant to that theme. Second, some students have used the short explanations that follow each answer as a guide to further reading and study. Finally, it is useful to try and compose scenarios or vignettes for all the items given in a list as another revision tool.

The EMQ format has evolved in the last 5 years. It is now generally accepted that a list of 10 possible answers with 5 scenarios is often not enough to provide enough distractors to produce challenging questions that will stretch the ablest of students. You may therefore face questions with more possible answers, fewer scenarios, or questions where each answer may be used more than once.

In this second edition, we have decided to keep the format unchanged but have added a further 50 questions. Some of these are at Distinction standard but we hope this will provide the stimulus required to encourage students to expand their depth of knowledge.

We hope you will learn as much from using this new edition as we did from writing it.

Cardiff   J.C.A.
2007   M.A.M.

Acknowledgements

We wish to thank all our colleagues who helped in the production of the first edition by reviewing the questions and making useful suggestions. These include Dr R. Alcolado, Dr M.D. Page, Dr N. Prasad, Dr A. Pandit, Dr K. Baboolal, Dr J. White, Dr J. Martin, Dr R. Dewar, Dr N. Robertson, Dr R. Dowdle, Dr P.S. Davies, Dr S. Aslan, Dr M. Edwards and Dr C. Long. In addition, we would like to thank Mr A. Ng for his input into many of the orthopaedic-themed questions that appear for the first time in this second edition.

Contents

Introduction

The assessment of medical students has been the subject of increasing scrutiny. While there is universal agreement that assessment or testing must be carried out, there are diverse opinions as to the best way to undertake this task. All agree that assessments should be fair, but the definition of fairness is elusive and too often in the past students have undergone assessments or examinations in which neither they nor their examiners were clear of the objectives.

The written examination in medicine has two important objectives. First, it is intended to identify students who have reached an acceptable academic and clinical standard. This is important to those entrusted with the training of doctors; they need to ensure that the examination is constructed in such a way that it covers the breadth and depth of knowledge they consider essential and that the marking is objective and reproducible. Second, a written examination provides an important learning experience for students. A properly constructed assessment can communicate to students what is more and what is less important; it can motivate them to read; and it can identify their areas of weakness for further study. This is the 'formative' as opposed to 'summative' role of examinations.

During its evolutionary process, the written examination has gone through the long essays, short notes, multiple-choice one-best-answer, and multiple-choice true/false/don't know item formats. The chief weakness of the long essay answers was that examinees could hide their areas of weakness by waffling around the subject, and by providing information that was not required but was vaguely germane to the question asked. The format is time-consuming to mark and suffered from the inevitable subjectivity of examiners. Students with good handwriting and grammar often score more highly than others with an equal or better knowledge of the subjects actually being assessed. The short-notes format forces students to concentrate on the specific question asked but, even with specific marking schedules, the problem of subjective judgement by examiners remains a major weakness.

The multiple-choice question (MCQ) format removed the examiners' subjectivity and provided a critical test of examinees' knowledge. During the last 50 years the MCQ formats have gone through various stages of scrutiny and in time, their flaws, or the flaws of those who set them, have come to the surface. Apart from technical flaws that give an advantage to test-wise examinees, this format tests recall of isolated facts and sometimes trivial knowledge without distinguishing it from the more important core knowledge. It is not good at testing clerking skills or the application of knowledge to clinical practice. The true/false dichotomy is poorly suited to medicine where most decisions require the integration of information and experience to reach what is considered the best option. A further problem is that with the passage of time, some of the wrong answers get merged with the right ones and are remembered as facts.

In the extended-matching format, each question is set around a theme that may be a symptom, sign, investigation, diagnosis or a management decision. This is followed by a clear, unambiguous lead-in statement asking the examinee to select an appropriate answer from a list of options, typically one for each of five extended 'stems' that describe a realistic clinical scenario. The questions are designed to test the application of knowledge to clinical assessment and management, by using patient vignettes relevant to clinical practice. These vignettes give details as encountered in clinical practice about patient's age, gender, occupation, history, relevant symptoms and signs and sometimes one or more key investigations. Although some of the options will be clearly very inappropriate (or 'false' in the traditional MCQ format), several might be possible and the student is asked to select the most appropriate or most likely for the scenario presented.

The extended-matching questions have their own problems and constraints. They are difficult and time-consuming to design. Each correct option should be the 'best' answer for its stem, and incorrect answers, or distracters, should be plausible and not deceptive or tricks. Sometimes the 'most likely' diagnosis will vary depending on the country from which the student has come and often the most important diagnosis to exclude in clinical practice will differ from the most common in pure epidemiological terms. The answers in the option list are placed in alphabetical order so as not to give test-wise students any unintended advantage. All new formats, guidelines and protocols become old in time and their hidden flaws emerge, and extended-match questions will be no exception. Despite these reservations, this format is worth adopting because it has considerable advantages over traditional multiple-choice papers. It has been in use for some years in the USA and is now being introduced in the UK.

THIS BOOK

All questions in this book are of the *standard extended-matching format*. They cover 150 key themes in medicine, surgery, obstetrics and gynaecology, paediatrics and psychiatry. Each themed question contains a list of 10 options from which have to be chosen the answers to five clinically realistic scenarios. Many cases are based on patients we have seen in our own practices. The complexity of the questions ranges from very easy to very difficult, with the majority of the questions lying in the middle of the knowledge spectrum.

We have included questions with a variety of forms, with both long and relatively short scenarios, to allow students to become familiar with the different types of question that may appear in examinations. The questions have been broadly divided into systems headings but, because medicine is not like this in practice, a third of the questions relate to important symptoms and signs. Although this book should give useful experience to both undergraduate and postgraduate students preparing for examinations, we believe that it can also provide a valuable learning experience to all students of clinical medicine. It contains 750 clinical scenarios, any of which a doctor may encounter in everyday practice, and as many decisions, some of which they may have to make every day.

USING THIS BOOK

We would suggest that students should read the lead-in statement carefully to understand what is required, and then study each stem without reference to the option list and generate their own answer for each stem. Finally, they should compare their answers with those given in the option list, and score 1 for each correct answer and 0 for the incorrect ones, there being no negative score in this format. It should be noted that in some types of extended-match examination, scoring is on a sliding scale with maximum marks for the best answer and negative marks if the answer given betrays a serious lack of understanding. Many examinations stipulate that any answer in the option list can be used once, more than once or not at all. In order to maximize the teaching potential of our questions, we have not used an answer more than once in any given question. This will help the reader with some questions (by a process of elimination) and therefore we estimate that an average undergraduate student should be able to score between 50% and 60%, and a very knowledgeable undergraduate or a postgraduate should score at least 75% on the questions in this book.

We have felt it particularly important to provide the reasoning for our answers after each question. These answers also contain other facts that may allow users to increase their knowledge as they work through the questions. In keeping with the objectives of formative assessment, it is more important to know why an answer is deemed right or wrong than the absolute numbers of correct answers attained in the assessment.

Unlike the more traditional multiple-choice format revision books, readers will find a place for this volume after the examination hurdle is passed. By using the index of themes, it will be possible to quickly look up a list of options that should be considered in clinical practice.

Key symptoms in clinical practice

ALTERED LEVEL OF CONSCIOUSNESS

1.1 **For each of the following patients with an altered level of consciousness, select the most likely diagnosis.**

A Brain stem infarction
B Drug overdose
C Hepatic failure
D Hypoglycaemia
E Hyponatraemia
F Hypothermia
G Meningitis
H Renal failure
I Schizophrenia
J Subarachnoid haemorrhage

1. A 92-year-old woman is admitted with an episode of collapse. Two days later, she remains deeply unconscious with pin-point pupils.

2. A 42-year-old man suddenly collapses. Fundoscopy reveals sub-hyaloid haemorrhages.

3. A 22-year-old woman is found collapsed on the street. On examination, she has pin-point pupils, is apyrexial and responds to painful stimuli.

4. A 46-year-old woman is found collapsed at home. On examination, she is unrousable, pyrexial and has a purpuric rash.

5. A 54-year-old man is found in a confused state. On examination, he has gynaecomastia and spider naevi. While being admitted to hospital he has a large haematemesis and becomes comatosed.

Answers to 1.1

1. **A. Brain stem infarction.** Pin-point pupils are commonly seen in patients who have suffered a brain-stem stroke. The brain stem is made up of the mid-brain, pons and medulla oblongata. Infarction in the region of the diencephalon will produce small, reactive pupils, though the pupils are so small that their reaction to light cannot be fully appreciated. Truly pin-point pupils occur in pontine haemorrhage and in opiate overdosage.

2. **J. Subarachnoid haemorrhage.** A sub-hyaloid haemorrhage has a characteristic sharply defined, rounded appearance. In the presence of a typical clinical scenario, it is pathognomonic of a subarachnoid haemorrhage.

3. **B. Drug overdose.** The patient is relatively young and although a number of the options are possible (e.g. subarachnoid), an opiate overdose would explain the pin-point pupils. The patient should be given an opiate antagonist such as Narcan and the response assessed.

4. **G. Meningitis.** A purpuric rash in a patient with neurological symptoms should suggest this diagnosis. Intravenous benzylpenicillin should be administered without further delay.

5. **C. Hepatic failure.** The patient has signs of chronic liver disease. The haematemesis may be due to bleeding oesophageal varices, a precipitant of hepatic encephalopathy.

DYSPHAGIA

1.2 **For each of the following patients with difficulty in swallowing, select the most likely cause.**

A   Achalasia
B   Arch aortic aneurysm
C   Benign peptic stricture
D   Carcinoma of the oesophagus
E   Foreign body
F   Guillain–Barré syndrome
G   Left atrial dilatation
H   Motor neurone disease
I   Pharyngeal pouch
J   Scleroderma

1. A 36-year-old man complains of difficulty in swallowing solids and liquids for the last 5 years. He has not lost any weight. His chest X-ray shows a fluid level within the mediastinum.

2. An 81-year-old woman complains of difficulty in eating her food. She tends to choke and has noticed a gurgling in her neck. When she lies in bed at night, she regurgitates some of the evening meal.

3. A 68-year-old woman complains of a 3-week history of difficulty in swallowing. Initially the problem was just with solid food but now it is with liquids as well. She has lost 6 kg in weight over the last 2 months.

4. A 79-year-old man who has needed to take antacids for many years complains of difficulty in swallowing that has been getting worse over the last 6 months. He thinks that he may have lost a few kg in weight.

5. A 50-year-old woman is admitted as an emergency with chest pain. She had been finishing a meal when the symptoms came on suddenly and she could not continue. She feels sick but cannot vomit, and on examination she is coughing up large quantities of saliva.

Answers to 1.2

1. **A. Achalasia.** The patient is relatively young and there is a long history but no weight loss. A characteristic feature of achalasia is difficulty in swallowing both liquids and solids from the onset of symptoms.

2. **I. Pharyngeal pouch.** Sensations of gurgling in the neck together with regurgitation of food in an elderly patient point to the correct diagnosis.

3. **D. Carcinoma of the oesophagus.** A relatively short history is common in patients with malignant disease in the oesophagus. There is rapid weight loss associated with progressive dysphagia.

4. **C. Benign peptic stricture.** The history is long, with years of previous dyspeptic symptoms. Unlike in oesophageal cancer, weight is well maintained.

5. **E. Foreign body.** This woman had swallowed a peach stone that completely obstructed the oesophagus and caused absolute dysphagia. She was unable to swallow her own saliva.

CHEST PAIN

1.3 **For each of the following patients with chest pain, select the most likely diagnosis.**

A   Angina
B   Anxiety
C   Dissecting aortic aneurysm
D   Lobar pneumonia
E   Myocardial infarction
F   Oesophagitis
G   Pericarditis
H   Pneumothorax
I   Pulmonary embolus
J   Tietze's syndrome

1. A 32-year-old man is admitted complaining of sudden-onset, severe, central chest pain that came on while bending over to lift a heavy box. The pain radiated down his back. The pain has now subsided but he complains of pins and needles in both lower limbs and he cannot stand. On examination, his blood pressure is 90/60 mmHg.

2. A 61-year-old woman visits her general practitioner complaining of chest pain and heaviness in her right arm when watching her favourite television 'soap'. The pain usually lasts 10 min before gradually subsiding. She also complains of shortness of breath when doing her gardening.

3. A 75-year-old woman visits her general practitioner complaining that 3 days previously, she had woken with central chest pain. The pain lasted all day but has now settled. However, since then she has developed a nocturnal cough and finds she is short of breath climbing her stairs.

4. A 40-year-old woman is admitted complaining of sudden-onset, sharp and severe chest pain. The pain is worse on movement and inspiration and she has a non-productive cough. On examination, her blood pressure is 90/40 mmHg, her jugular venous pressure (JVP) is raised 7 cm but examination of the chest is unremarkable.

5. A 40-year-old man is admitted complaining of sudden-onset, sharp and severe chest pain. The pain is worse on inspiration. On examination, he is tachycardic and tachypnoeic, the trachea is central but there is reduced chest expansion on the left associated with hyper-resonance on percussion and reduced breath sounds.

Answers to 1.3

1. **C. Dissecting aortic aneurysm.** Sudden-onset chest pain while lifting is commonly musculoskeletal in origin or due to gastro-oesophageal reflux. However, this patient is hypotensive and has neurological signs in the lower limbs. A dissecting thoracic aortic aneurysm is the only diagnosis in the list given that can unify all these features.

2. **A. Angina.** The pain of angina may come on at 'rest', especially if the patient is stressed or aroused, e.g. watching a television programme. Often patients describe the sensation as difficulty in breathing and, if this occurs regularly on exertion, a diagnosis of angina should be considered. Although a myocardial infarction may have occurred, the history of a brief episode of pain is more of chronic stable angina.

3. **E. Myocardial infarction.** Central chest pain waking a patient from sleep is a relatively common presentation of a myocardial infarction. Other causes are possible, but this patient subsequently develops symptoms suggestive of cardiac failure, making infarction more likely than simple angina.

4. **I. Pulmonary embolus.** The patient has pleuritic chest pain. The raised jugular venous pressure suggests right-sided heart failure and, together with hypotension, makes the diagnosis of a pulmonary embolus more likely than the other causes of chest pain. Chest examination is frequently normal in patients, even if they have a life-threatening pulmonary embolus.

5. **H. Pneumothorax.** The symptoms suggest a respiratory cause for the chest pain. Although a pulmonary embolus or pneumonia should be considered, the hyper-resonance and reduced breath sounds places a pneumothorax at the top of the differential diagnosis. The trachea is deviated only in a large pneumothorax under significant tension, causing displacement of the mediastinum.

SUDDEN-ONSET SHORTNESS OF BREATH

1.4 **For each of the following patients who present with sudden-onset shortness of breath, select the most likely diagnosis.**

A   Acute exacerbation of chronic obstructive pulmonary disease (COPD)
B   Acute pulmonary oedema
C   Acute severe asthma
D   Anaphylaxis
E   Inhaled foreign body
F   Lobar collapse
G   Metabolic acidosis
H   Pneumonia
I   Pneumothorax
J   Pulmonary embolus

1. A 35-year-old woman presents complaining of sudden-onset, severe shortness of breath associated with sharp chest pain. She is a smoker and is on the oral contraceptive pill. On examination, the trachea is central, chest expansion is symmetrically decreased, percussion note is normal, there are decreased breath sounds and a pleural rub over the left mid-zone.

2. A 32-year-old man is suddenly taken ill in a restaurant with shortness of breath. He is a heavy smoker. On examination, he has stridor, the trachea is central and there is globally reduced air entry with excessive supraclavicular recession.

3. A 19-year-old woman presents to her general practitioner complaining of shortness of breath and tight bilateral chest pain. She is a smoker and is on the oral contraceptive pill. On examination, the trachea is central, the chest appears hyperinflated, percussion note is resonant throughout and there is scattered expiratory wheeze.

4. The wife of a 60-year-old man calls an ambulance because he has woken at 3 a.m. with severe shortness of breath. By the time he reaches hospital he looks grey and sweaty. His trachea is central, percussion note is resonant and there are widespread inspiratory crackles and wheeze.

5. A 16-year-old man is found in a semi-conscious state, breathing heavily. He is a non-smoker. Apart from his breathing, chest examination is normal as are his chest X-ray and ECG.

Answers to 1.4

1. **J. Pulmonary embolus.** The main differential diagnosis here lies between pneumonia and pulmonary embolus. They both can produce decreased breath sounds and a pleural rub. The sudden onset of the pain, the normal percussion note and lack of crackles, make a pulmonary embolus more likely.

2. **E. Inhaled foreign body.** Stridor is a sign of large airways obstruction. A large inhaled foreign body causes immediate symptoms and the proximal obstruction due to the foreign body is the cause of the globally reduced air entry. Smaller bodies may present with intermittent bouts of coughing, especially in children.

3. **C. Acute severe asthma.** Hyperinflated lungs should always suggest the diagnosis of asthma or chronic small airways disease. Although most patients will have audible wheeze, in severe asthma, the chest may become almost silent as a result of the poor air entry. Chest pain is a common symptom in patients with asthma. It is sometimes difficult clinically to exclude a pulmonary embolus in a patient with known asthma who presents with chest pain and shortness of breath.

4. **B. Acute pulmonary oedema.** This scenario is a common medical emergency. Intravenous diamorphine or furosemide (frusemide) results in a rapid improvement. Wheeze may be a predominant feature in cardiac failure ('cardiac asthma'), but responds to diuretics rather than nebulized bronchodilators which may exacerbate underlying cardiac ischaemia.

5. **G. Metabolic acidosis.** Kussmaul's respiration is the term applied to the deep breathing of patients with a metabolic acidosis. It causes a reduction in the P_{CO_2} and helps to buffer the acidosis. Common causes are diabetic ketoacidosis and severe aspirin overdose. Not all patients who appear short of breath have a cardiopulmonary cause.

SHORTNESS OF BREATH

1.5   **For each of the following patients who present with shortness of breath, select the most likely diagnosis.**

A   Acute respiratory distress syndrome
B   Asbestosis
C   Asthma
D   Complex pneumoconiosis
E   Cryptogenic fibrosing alveolitis
F   Progressive massive fibrosis
G   Sarcoidosis
H   Siderosis
I   Simple coal workers' pneumoconiosis
J   Tuberculosis

1.   A 59-year-old ex-miner gives a history of gradually increasing shortness of breath and melanoptysis. On examination, he is centrally cyanosed, has bilateral ankle swelling and a raised jugular venous pressure. Auscultation of the chest reveals inspiratory crackles and wheezes. His chest X-ray shows widespread fibrosis with confluent areas affecting > 30% of the lung fields and cavitation in the upper lobes.

2.   A 56-year-old ex-miner attends the chest clinic for a routine review. He says that on a good day he can walk around 300 m before becoming short of breath. He has a chronic cough productive of small amounts of yellow sputum. On examination, he is not cyanosed but does have mild ankle swelling. The jugular venous pulse is just visible when he is lying flat. The chest X-ray shows patchy fibrosis and nodules between 1 and 3 mm in diameter.

3.   A 52-year-old ex-miner complains of episodes of shortness of breath. The attacks are generally worse in the morning and in dusty atmospheres. In between attacks, he has no symptoms and examination is normal. His chest X-ray shows hyperexpanded lungs but no other abnormalities.

4.   A 38-year-old arc-welder reports increasing shortness of breath over the last 12 months at his regular occupational medical examination. Examination is unremarkable but a chest X-ray shows fine nodules spread throughout the lung fields with no associated fibrosis.

5.   A 65-year-old ex-shipyard worker is admitted to hospital with symptoms of a respiratory tract infection. His chest X-ray shows patchy fibrosis and linear pleural plaques.

Answers to 1.5

1. **F. Progressive massive fibrosis.** Melanoptysis is the coughing up of black sputum. Cavitation of the upper lobes may be due to reactivation of tuberculosis in the damaged lung. There is progressive right-sided heart failure.

2. **I. Simple coal workers' pneumoconiosis.** The pulmonary fibrosis will not progress now that the patient has left the mining industry. However, co-existent emphysema and chronic bronchitis may deteriorate over time.

3. **C. Asthma.** The patient has paroxysmal shortness of breath typical of asthma. Asthma may appear for the first time in middle age. Given the occupational history, lung function tests would be useful to distinguish the obstructive picture of asthma from the restrictive picture of fibrosis.

4. **H. Siderosis.** Iron oxide is deposited in the lung resulting in the chest X-ray findings. There is no associated fibrosis and an alternative cause for the shortness of breath should be sought.

5. **B. Asbestosis.** Pleural plaques suggest previous asbestos exposure and the substance was used widely in shipbuilding. The patient is at increased risk of both squamous cell carcinoma of the bronchus and mesothelioma.

HAEMOPTYSIS

1.6 **For each of the following patients with haemoptysis, select the most likely diagnosis.**

A   Acute bronchitis
B   Acute left ventricular failure
C   Bronchial adenoma
D   Bronchiectasis
E   Carcinoma
F   Goodpasture's syndrome
G   Lung abscess
H   Mitral stenosis
I   Pulmonary infarction
J   Tuberculosis (TB)

1.   A 70-year-old man complains of recurrent bouts of coughing up sputum with small streaks of blood. The chest X-ray shows reduced volume of the left lung field.

2.   A 62-year-old man complains of sudden-onset shortness of breath associated with sharp chest pain, worse on inspiration or movement. He has coughed up teaspoon-sized quantities of dark red blood. His chest X-ray shows linear atelectasis at the left base and a small pleural effusion.

3.   A 36-year-old man had a flu-like illness last week and then started coughing up blood. On the day of his admission to hospital, he noticed that his urine looks dark and 'smoky'. He is mildly short of breath and has bilateral ankle swelling. His chest X-ray shows diffuse intra-alveolar shadowing and dip-stick testing of his urine confirms haematuria.

4.   A 58-year-old woman attends her general practitioner complaining of increasing shortness of breath. In particular, she has been waking short of breath at night when she coughs up frothy pink sputum. The chest X-ray shows intra-alveolar shadowing and upper lobe blood vessel diversion.

5.   A 48-year-old man complains of coughing up blood occasionally over the last 2 months. He is a smoker and had whooping cough as a child. For several years, he has been coughing up large quantities of sputum, especially in the winter months. While awaiting his out-patient appointment, he has a massive haemoptysis that requires urgent admission. His chest X-ray shows an enlarged cardiac outline, hyperinflated lungs with prominent peribronchial markings.

Answers to 1.6

1. **E. Carcinoma.** Streaks of blood in the sputum suggest the source of bleeding is in the bronchial tree rather than the mouth or pharynx. The chest X-ray finding is suggestive of a left main bronchus tumour.

2. **I. Pulmonary infarction.** The history is highly suggestive of a pulmonary embolus. Haemoptysis in this condition may range from none to massive. Typically, the patient coughs up frank blood rather than blood-stained sputum. The chest X-ray findings are in keeping with the diagnosis. Occasionally, the classic 'wedge-shaped' pulmonary infarct can be seen, although more often the X-ray is either normal or shows atelectasis.

3. **F. Goodpasture's syndrome.** Pulmonary haemorrhage with associated haematuria should always raise the possibility of Goodpasture's. This is a disease of males (6:1 male to female ratio) characterized by the triad of pulmonary haemorrhage, glomerulonephritis and anti-glomerular basement membrane antibody.

4. **B. Acute left ventricular failure.** Pink, frothy sputum is typical of pulmonary oedema.

5. **D. Bronchiectasis.** The history of large quantities of sputum should raise the suspicion of bronchiectasis. Childhood pneumonias such as pertussis and measles are recognized risk factors. Recurrent small haemoptysis is frequent but patients may also suffer large, life-threatening episodes.

VOMITING

1.7 **In each of the following patients presenting with vomiting, select the most likely diagnosis.**

A   Acute pancreatitis
B   Carcinoma of the oesophagus
C   Cerebral tumour
D   Duodenal atresia
E   Gastrocolic fistula
F   Meningitis
G   Peptic ulcer
H   Pyloric stenosis
I   Renal failure
J   Viral gastroenteritis

1. A 5-week-old first-born baby boy has been vomiting for over a week. His progress was quite satisfactory for the first 3 weeks but since then he has had vomiting which has become persistent and he is now losing weight. His mother says that he vomits soon after the feed and it jets out with some force. On examination, he has a sunken anterior fontanelle.

2. A 38-year-old electrician with a past history of Crohn's disease presents with persistent vomiting and abdominal pain of 10 hours' duration. His vomitus has an unpleasant smell and on close examination shows faecal material. He is dehydrated with a tachycardia and low blood pressure.

3. A 2-week-old neonate boy has been vomiting since birth. Initially there was some spilling of his feed but the vomiting has become persistent and it contains greenish fluid suggestive of bile.

4. A 22-year-old student has been feeling generally unwell and feverish for a couple of days. For the last 10 h he has developed a headache and he has vomited three times which came without any warning nausea.

5. A 42-year-old bank manager has had an upper abdominal pain for about 6 months. He put up with it but during the last 3 days he has vomited five times and each time he brought up coffee ground fluid mixed up with some undigested food.

Answers to 1.7

1. **H. Pyloric stenosis – *projectile vomiting.*** Pyloric stenosis is most common in first-born male children and vomiting usually starts any time between the 3rd and 6th week. The projectile character suggests the diagnosis. The diagnosis can often be made by observing a feeding experience when a swelling of about 2 cm diameter may be seen and felt as a firm mass in the region of the neonate's pylorus.

2. **E. Gastrocolic fistula – *faeculent vomiting.*** The past history of Crohn's disease is helpful but it is the presence of faecal material in the vomitus which suggests the presence of a communication between the large bowel and the stomach or duodenum. An obstruction of the lower ileum or large bowel may also lead to faeculent vomiting.

3. **D. Duodenal atresia – *bile in the vomitus.*** The presence of bile in the vomitus of a neonate, who starts vomiting soon after birth, is a serious sign. The other possible causes of obstruction are a band, midgut volvulus, meconium ileus and an annular pancreas. If untreated, any of these conditions will progress to perforation and infarction of the gut.

4. **F. Meningitis – *neurogenic/central vomiting.*** The vomiting caused by meningitis or intracranial hypertension due to any cause is not preceded by nausea unless there is coincident upper gut disease. The patient may sometimes volunteer that the first vomiting took him by surprise as it came out of the blue. In this case, the history is more suggestive of meningitis than a cerebral tumour.

5. **G. Peptic ulcer – *coffee ground vomiting.*** This is a fairly straightforward presentation of peptic ulcer disease. The 'coffee grounds' are specks of altered blood.

UPPER ABDOMINAL PAIN

1.8 **For each of the following clinical presentations, match the most likely diagnosis from the list.**

A Acute cholecystitis
B Ampullary carcinoma
C Benign stricture of the bile duct
D Carcinoma of the bile duct
E Carcinoma of the gall bladder
F Choledocholithiasis
G Chronic cholecystitis
H Peptic ulcer disease
I Typhoid cholecystitis
J Unstable angina

1. A 46-year-old housewife was woken up at 3 a.m. by a severe pain in the right upper abdomen and below the right shoulder blade. She was restless, vomited twice and felt hot and sweaty. She had a temperature of 39°C and had tenderness, guarding and rigidity in the right hypochondrium.

2. A 50-year-old district nurse had recurrent episodes of pain in right upper quadrant of her abdomen for 3 weeks. During the last week, she felt unwell with malaise, sweating, rigors and generalized itching and was alarmed to notice that she was passing dark urine and pale stools. Her doctor found that she was mildly jaundiced and febrile but that there were no palpable masses in the abdomen.

3. A 55-year-old school cleaner had a long history of abdominal pain and was awaiting a cholecystectomy. While she was waiting for the operation, her pain became persistent, she lost 4 kg in weight and her friend told her that she looked like a buttercup. Her doctor could feel a mass in the right hypochondrium.

4. A 45-year-old housewife had two episodes of upper abdominal pain during the previous 6 months. A week ago, she saw her doctor because of a pain in the right subcostal region, which radiated to the back of the right chest. A cholecystogram showed a non-functioning gall bladder.

5. A 48-year-old general practitioner had two episodes of a burning sensation in the epigastrium. He took some antacids and took his dog out for a walk to get some fresh air but felt his stomach tightening up. He went to bed early but was woken by a burning sensation in his oesophagus, which radiated to his jaw. He was breathless, cold and clammy.

Answers to 1.8

1. **A. Acute cholecystitis.** This is a typical presentation of acute cholecystitis. Females are affected three times more often than males. Although it is usually said that patients with acute cholecystitis are females, flabby and over 40, no age is exempt. There is often a history of similar episodes. The pain is often referred to the tip of the right shoulder and to the right infrascapular region. Jaundice is rare in uncomplicated cases.

2. **F. Choledocholithiasis.** The jaundice, pruritus, dark urine and pale stools all suggest bile duct obstruction. The gall bladder is usually impalpable in accordance with Courvoisier's law, which states that in obstructive jaundice a palpable, distended gall bladder is not the result of gallstones. In choledocholithiasis, the gall bladder is usually shrunken from cholecystitis. A painless increasing jaundice with a palpable gall bladder suggests the presence of a neoplasm.

3. **E. Carcinoma of the gall bladder.** Females are affected more commonly than men in a ratio of 4:1. A palpable gall bladder in a patient with a history of gallstones is an ominous finding suggestive of a carcinoma of the gall bladder. Weight loss and progressive jaundice are additional pointers to a neoplastic cause.

4. **B. Chronic cholecystitis.** Recurrent attacks of acute cholecystitis, which vary in severity, usually progress to chronic cholecystitis. The differential diagnosis is from peptic ulcer disease, hiatus hernia, angina, carcinoma of the stomach and renal calculi though chronic cholecystitis may co-exist with any one of them. The presence of gallstones or a non-functioning gall bladder is highly suggestive of chronic cholecystitis.

5. **J. Unstable angina.** This is an important diagnosis to be borne in mind when considering a history of epigastric burning sensation or pain, which does not respond to antacids and returns in a cluster of attacks. The story would also be consistent with acute myocardial infarction, which was not on the list. The association of breathlessness and cold and clammy peripheries strongly point to a cardiac cause of his epigastric burning sensation.

ABDOMINAL PAIN I

1.9 **For each of the following patients with abdominal pain, select the most likely diagnosis.**

Normal value; amylase <150 IU.

A   Acute pancreatitis
B   Appendicitis
C   Biliary colic
D   Diverticulitis
E   Hypochondriasis
F   Perforated peptic ulcer
G   Pyelonephritis
H   Ruptured aortic aneurysm
I   Salpingitis
J   Ureteric colic

1. A 17-year-old woman is admitted complaining of vomiting and lower abdominal pain. She is tender in the right iliac fossa. The urine dip-stick test is normal. The serum amylase is 90 IU.

2. A 19-year-old woman is admitted with vomiting and lower abdominal pain. She is tender in the right loin. The urine dip-stick tests shows blood +++ and protein +. The serum amylase is 200 IU.

3. A 51-year-old man is admitted with vomiting and sudden-onset epigastric pain. On examination, the abdomen is rigid. The urine dip-stick test shows no blood but a trace of protein. An abdominal X-ray shows a loop of dilated small bowel in the epigastrium and the serum calcium is 1.9 mmol/L.

4. A 22-year-old man is admitted with vomiting and abdominal pain. On examination, the abdomen is rigid and bowel sounds are absent. The urine dip-stick test is normal and the serum amylase is 150 IU.

5. An 82-year-old woman is admitted with vomiting and abdominal pain. On examination, she is tender in the left iliac fossa with guarding and rebound tenderness. The urine dip-stick test shows a trace of blood but not protein and the serum amylase is 75 IU.

Answers to 1.9

1. **B. Acute appendicitis.** The other possibilities include pyelonephritis (but the urine dip-stick test is normal) and salpingitis. Although the latter must be considered, no history is given of other gynaecological symptoms and appendicitis is a more likely diagnosis.

2. **G. Pyelonephritis.** The tender loin and urine dip-stick result suggest a renal cause for the symptoms. Ureteric colic is unlikely, since the pain is not characteristic of this disorder and renal stones would also be uncommon in a woman of this age. Blood and protein in the urine are a feature of urinary tract infection and not necessarily of renal stones.

3. **A. Acute pancreatitis.** Sudden-onset epigastric pain, vomiting and rigidity of the abdomen are suggestive of acute pancreatitis. The presence of a loop of dilated small bowel near the pancreas ('sentinel loop') is also characteristic. *Note* that a low serum calcium is a poor prognostic factor. The serum amylase in this case was 1500 IU.

4. **F. Perforated peptic ulcer.** This is seen less often now than in the past, perhaps related to the increased use of potent ulcer-healing drugs such as the proton pump inhibitors. The amylase is normal and the normal urine dip-stick test makes a renal cause for the presentation unlikely. Late presentation of acute appendicitis could result in this picture but this patient with signs of peritonitis in fact had a perforated duodenal ulcer.

5. **D. Diverticulitis.** The symptoms and signs of 'left-sided appendicitis' are characteristic of acute diverticulitis.

ABDOMINAL PAIN II

1.10 For each of the following patients with abdominal pain, select the most likely cause.

A   Acute cholecystitis
B   Aortic aneurysm
C   Biliary colic
D   Crohn's disease
E   Diverticulitis
F   Duodenal ulcer
G   Intussusception
H   Pancreatitis
I   Pyelonephritis
J   Sigmoid volvulus

1.   A 77-year-old man is transferred to hospital from an 'Elderly Mentally Infirm' Unit with sudden colicky lower abdominal pain. His carers say that he has suffered from chronic constipation and intermittent rectal bleeding. On examination, the abdomen is distended and tender. A plain X-ray shows dilated large bowel and the caecum is visible in the right lower quadrant.

2.   A 22-year-old man is admitted urgently to hospital complaining of severe central abdominal pain. Initially the pain was colicky but has become constant. He has vomited and has passed dark red blood per rectum. He has recently been investigated for iron deficiency anaemia.

3.   A 38-year-old woman is admitted to hospital with vomiting and severe upper abdominal pain going through to her back. She gives a 6-month history of fatty food intolerance and intermittent right upper quadrant pain and a recent ultrasound confirmed she had gallstones. On examination, the abdomen is rigid. The corrected serum calcium is 1.8 mmol/L.

4.   A 76-year-old woman is admitted to hospital in a confused state. On examination, she is dehydrated and complains of colicky left-sided lower abdominal pain. On examination, there is rebound tenderness in the left iliac fossa.

5.   A 35-year-old man is admitted to hospital with severe upper abdominal pain. The pain comes in waves, each lasting a few minutes. He is unable to get comfortable in the bed and is clutching his right hypochondrium. The serum amylase is just above the upper limit of normal.

Answers to 1.10

1. **J. Sigmoid volvulus.** An enlarged loop of sigmoid colon has twisted on its mesentery to cause symptoms. The condition is rare in the USA and Western Europe but cases are reported in patients living in institutions, presumably because chronic constipation and dilatation of the sigmoid colon predispose to volvulus. In younger patients, the presentation is similar to that of any other abdominal catastrophe but in elderly patients, a subacute form may present with intermittent symptoms, although bowel infarction may supervene with abdominal pain, constipation and rectal bleeding. The X-ray findings support the diagnosis. Similar symptoms may be caused by a caecal volvulus but then the caecum is not visible in its normal position in the right lower quadrant.

2. **G. Intussusception.** The vast majority of these occur in childhood. This patient had an inverted Meckel's diverticulum causing his iron deficiency anaemia and this predisposed to intussusception in adult life. The symptoms of abdominal cramps, nausea and rectal bleeding are episodic as the intussusception comes and goes.

3. **H. Pancreatitis.** Gallstones are a major risk factor for the development of acute pancreatitis. Although a serum amylase should be requested, a low serum calcium supports the diagnosis and is a marker of the severity of the attack. The level of calcium in the serum is thought to fall as a result of sequestration of calcium in areas of intraperitoneal fat necrosis. A concentration below 1.8 mmol/L is a poor prognostic sign.

4. **E. Diverticulitis.** This may present as 'left-sided appendicitis'. *Note* that elderly patients may be too unwell to give a coherent history and there are many possible causes of dehydration and confusion. A careful physical examination is essential if important diagnoses are not to be missed.

5. **C. Biliary colic.** The clinical picture is typical of a patient passing biliary stones through the bile duct. The bilirubin and amylase may be moderately raised but this is not invariably the case.

HAEMATEMESIS

1.11 For each of the following patients with haematemesis, select the most likely diagnosis.

A   Barrett's oesophagus
B   Carcinoma of the duodenum
C   Carcinoma of stomach
D   Gastric erosions
E   Mallory–Weiss tear
F   Oesophageal varices
G   Oesophagitis
H   Peptic ulcer
I   Pharyngeal pouch
J   Vascular malformations

1.   A 52-year-old man is admitted to hospital following a haematemesis. His family is concerned that he has lost a lot of weight recently. On examination, there is a mass in the epigastrium and enlarged supraclavicular lymph nodes.

2.   A 36-year-old woman is admitted following a haematemesis. She has had at least four previous admissions with GI haemorrhage. On examination, there are small pigmented lesions around her lips.

3.   A 19-year-old man is air-lifted from a North Sea cruise liner following a large haematemesis that followed a prolonged period of sea-sickness.

4.   A 32-year-old man is admitted in a collapsed state after being found in a pool of blood. In hospital, he continues to have massive haematemesis. On examination, he has gynaecomastia and spider naevi. There is no hepatosplenomegaly and he says that he drinks alcohol only socially.

5.   A 60-year-old man is admitted to hospital following a road traffic accident. He is managed on the Intensive Care Unit but you are called to see him after they observe blood in the nasogastric aspirate.

Answers to 1.11

1. **C. Carcinoma of the stomach.** The mass in the epigastrium and supraclavicular lymph nodes make malignancy likely. Carcinoma of the duodenum is very rare.

2. **J. Vascular malformations.** This woman has Peutz–Jeghers syndrome. The pigmented lesions around the lips are associated with intestinal polyposis and vascular malformations.

3. **E. Mallory–Weiss tear.** Commonly seen after recurrent vomiting from alcohol ingestion, a tear of the oesophageal mucosa may be caused by severe vomiting due to motion sickness. Although often considered trivial, it should be noted that life-threatening blood loss may occur.

4. **F. Oesophageal varices.** The patient has signs of chronic liver disease and varices may have developed as a result of portal hypertension. In alcoholic liver disease, the liver is often small and not palpable and the spleen may not be palpable after a large haematemesis, even if it is normally enlarged. A history of 'social' drinking is unhelpful, since it gives no information about the absolute alcohol intake. The haematemesis is described as 'massive' and this makes oesophageal varices the most likely correct answer. However, it should be noted that many patients with known varices are actually bleeding from a peptic ulcer since the two frequently co-exist.

5. **D. Gastric erosions.** Superficial erosions may develop during acute illnesses and many Intensive Care Units use proton pump inhibitors or sucralfate in an attempt to reduce their occurrence.

LOWER GASTROINTESTINAL HAEMORRHAGE

1.12 **For each of the following patients presenting with a lower gastrointestinal haemorrhage, select the most likely diagnosis.**

A   Anal fissure
B   Angiodysplasia
C   Carcinoma of the colon
D   Coeliac disease
E   Crohn's disease
F   Diverticular disease
G   Ischaemia
H   Meckel's diverticulum
I   Solitary rectal ulcer
J   Ulcerative colitis

1.   A 72-year-old woman is admitted to hospital following profuse, dark red, rectal bleeding. On examination, she is hypotensive and has a tachycardia. She gives a history of recurrent left iliac fossa pain and constipation over the last 5–10 years but otherwise she has been well.

2.   A 71-year-old woman is admitted to hospital following profuse, dark red, rectal bleeding. On examination, she is hypotensive and tachycardic. She was admitted with a similar episode 4 months previously, and at that time a barium enema was reported as normal. The bleeding stops spontaneously. A colonoscopy is performed and this shows multiple small dark red spots on the mucosa.

3.   A 13-year-old girl is admitted to hospital following profuse rectal bleeding. She has had three similar episodes in the last year. Previous investigations have included a barium enema and colonoscopy, both of which were normal.

4.   A 48-year-old man, who has been previously fit and well, visits his general practitioner because he has noticed bright red blood on the toilet paper after wiping himself. This has been associated with pain when opening his bowels.

5.   A 47-year-old man, who has been previously fit and well, visits his general practitioner because he has noticed some dark red blood mixed in with his stools. He has been going to the toilet more often recently but otherwise feels well.

Answers to 1.12

1. **F. Diverticular disease.** The history is not suggestive of inflammatory bowel disease, anal fissure or a solitary rectal ulcer. Coeliac disease is not a cause of lower GI haemorrhage. Of the remaining possibilities, a brisk haemorrhage from diverticular disease is the most likely. Angiodysplasia is relatively rare and a Meckel's diverticulum haemorrhage even rarer. Carcinoma of the colon is likely to present with altered bowel habit or more insidious bleeding. Constipation and a nagging left lower quadrant pain are important features of diverticular disease. There is no mention of abdominal distension or tenderness as may have been expected in ischaemic colitis, although this is probably the next best answer.

2. **B. Angiodysplasia.** This is a disease of the elderly where vascular malformations develop, usually in the right side of the colon. It is a relatively common cause of anaemia of obscure cause but many patients probably remain undiagnosed despite numerous investigations. Angiography is the procedure of choice in these cases.

3. **H. Meckel's diverticulum.** Although this patient is young, a Meckel's diverticulum may first present in elderly patients. Peptic ulceration in the ileal mucosa (from unbuffered secretions from the ectopic gastric mucosa) and intestinal obstruction (due to volvulus or intussusception) are two major complications (others include perforation, enteritis and neoplasia) of a Meckel's diverticulum. The haemorrhage from ectopic peptic ulcers is usually bright red, occasionally black and tarry but almost never occult.

4. **A. Anal fissure.** Bright red blood on the toilet paper suggests a local cause. The fissure may have been caused by constipation or local trauma. It may also be a sign of underlying Crohn's disease.

5. **C. Carcinoma of the colon.** Blood mixed with the stool is a worrying symptom. Tenesmus refers to the desire to pass stool even when a motion has recently occurred. It can be due to a rectal carcinoma or polyp.

RECTAL BLEEDING

1.13 **For each of the following patients presenting with rectal bleeding, select the most likely cause.**

A   Adenomatous rectal polyp
B   Anal fissure
C   Angiodysplasia
D   Carcinoma of the anus
E   Diverticular disease
F   Haemorrhoids
G   Ischaemic colitis
H   Meckel's diverticulum
I   Solitary rectal ulcer
J   Ulcerative colitis

1. A 45-year-old man complains of a 1-week history of pain on passing stool. The pain is severe and lasts for up to 1 h after passing the stool. He has also noticed bright red blood on the toilet paper after wiping himself.

2. A 42-year-old woman complains of a several-year history of intermittent bright red blood on the toilet paper after wiping herself. Clinically, she appears otherwise well and rectal examination is normal.

3. A 68-year-old woman presents with a 1-week history of diarrhoea. She is opening her bowels several times an hour during the day and up to 10 times during the night. She is passing unformed stool containing mucus and blood.

4. An 80-year-old man is admitted to hospital in a shocked state. On examination, his pulse is 120/min, blood pressure 90/60 mmHg and his abdomen appears generally distended and tender. He is passing small quantities of dark red blood per rectum.

5. A 79-year-old woman is admitted to hospital after passing a large quantity of bright red blood per rectum. By the time she arrives, the bleeding has stopped. Rectal examination is normal apart from blood on the finger and she complains of some tenderness in the left iliac fossa.

Answers to 1.13

1.   **B. Anal fissure.** This is the most locally painful of the
     conditions listed. The trauma of passing stool will open up the
     anal fissure and cause further pain. Haemorrhoids are not
     painful unless they become thrombosed.

2.   **F. Haemorrhoids.** Intermittent rectal bleeding is often the only
     symptom. The history is of several years and the patient is
     otherwise well, making more sinister causes of rectal bleeding
     unlikely (although they should still be excluded). Internal
     haemorrhoids are not palpable on rectal examination.

3.   **J. Ulcerative colitis.** The main differential diagnosis here is an
     infective colitis producing bloody diarrhoea (dysentery).

4.   **G. Ischaemic colitis.** Although bleeding from diverticular
     disease, Meckel's and angiodysplasia can be severe enough to
     produce circulatory shock. In this man, the degree of shock
     seems disproportionate to the amount of haemorrhage. This is
     due to the presence of infarcted bowel. The diagnosis is not
     uncommonly missed and should be considered in any elderly
     patient who suddenly develops abdominal pain and rectal
     bleeding.

5.   **E. Diverticular disease.** Angiodysplasia and a Meckel's
     diverticulum are possible, but less likely causes in a woman of
     this age.

DIARRHOEA

1.14 **For each of the following patients, select the most likely cause for their diarrhoea.**

A Autonomic dysfunction
B Coeliac disease
C Crohn's disease
D Cystic fibrosis
E Glucagonoma
F Ischaemic colitis
G Lymphoma
H Tropical sprue
I Ulcerative colitis
J Whipple's disease

1. A 16-year-old man presents with diarrhoea. He is opening his bowels at least 10 times a night and 20 times during the day, passing blood and scanty mucus. He has generalized abdominal pain and tenderness. Colonoscopy reveals confluent inflammatory lesions throughout most of the colon and biopsies are reported as showing crypt abscesses.

2. A 79-year-old woman presents in a collapsed state, passing bright red blood per rectum. On examination, she is shocked and her abdomen is distended and tender. Colonoscopy shows a haemorrhagic mucosa and the biopsies show marked necrosis and numerous inflammatory cells.

3. A 52-year-old man is seen by his general practitioner complaining of episodic left iliac fossa pain, flushing attacks and diarrhoea. On examination, he has an erythematous rash on his trunk, arms and face. A colonoscopy is normal.

4. An 18-year-old woman presents to the endocrine clinic with short stature and delayed puberty. She has suffered from recurrent abdominal bloating and loose motions for several years. On examination, she is thin and has signs of early puberty. Initial investigations show her to have an iron deficiency anaemia. Both upper and lower gastrointestinal endoscopies appear normal but duodenal biopsies show villous atrophy.

5. A 48-year-old man presents with recurrent abdominal bloating, loose motions and joint pains for several years. On examination, he is thin, pigmented and looks unwell. Initial investigations show him to have an iron deficiency anaemia. Both upper and lower gastrointestinal endoscopies appear normal but duodenal biopsies show the presence of particles that stain with PAS.

Answers to 1.14

1. **I. Ulcerative colitis.** Crypt abscesses are a typical feature in biopsies of the affected mucosa. The history given is typical of an acute episode of ulcerative colitis. In some cases, it may be difficult to distinguish a first episode from an infective colitis, e.g. salmonella.

2. **F. Ischaemic colitis.** This diagnosis should be suspected in any elderly patient who suddenly develops rectal bleeding. Unlike ulcerative colitis, biopsies show necrosis and no crypt abscesses. Barium enema may show characteristic narrowing of the bowel lumen with 'thumbprints' in the wall.

3. **E. Glucagonoma.** Recurrent attacks of diarrhoea in a patient complaining of flushing attacks or with a generalized skin rash should suggest the possibility of an endocrine cause. The diagnosis may be confirmed by measuring serum levels of gut peptides.

4. **B. Coeliac disease.** Malabsorption syndromes should always be considered in patients presenting with short stature and delayed puberty. Positive anti-endomysial antibodies may help to make the diagnosis but co-existent IgA deficiency in some patients means that the antibodies will not be present.

5. **J. Whipple's disease.** Abdominal pain, steatorrhoea and diffuse pigmentation in a middle-aged patient should raise the suspicion of Whipple's disease. The presence of PAS-positive particles in the duodenal biopsies are diagnostic of the condition. Multi-system involvement results in arthropathy, pancarditis and neurological deficits.

COLLAPSE

1.15 **For each of the following patients admitted after an episode of collapse, select the most likely diagnosis.**

A   Aortic stenosis
B   Carotid sinus hypersensitivity
C   Complete heart block
D   Epilepsy
E   Hypertrophic obstructive cardiomyopathy
F   Hyperventilation syndrome
G   Postural hypotension
H   Pulmonary embolus
I   Simple faint (vasovagal attack)
J   Ventricular tachycardia

1. A 21-year-old man collapses while playing football. When he regains consciousness, he feels well and denies any chest pain. There are no neurological signs but there is an ejection systolic murmur at the left sternal edge. His lying blood pressure is 110/70 mmHg.

2. A 17-year-old woman complains of feeling unwell while visiting her father in hospital. She collapses to the ground and looks pale and sweaty. Her pulse is 52 bpm and regular, and her lying blood pressure is 100/60 mmHg.

3. An 82-year-old woman with long-standing type 2 diabetes and hypertension says that over the last few months she has had attacks of light-headedness, especially on getting out of bed in the mornings. Her lying blood pressure is 100/60 mmHg.

4. A 77-year-old man collapses while out shopping. On regaining consciousness, he complains of some chest pain. In the last year, he has had several other episodes of collapse and chest pain on exertion. His lying blood pressure is 120/95 mmHg and he has an ejection systolic murmur at the left sternal edge that radiates into the neck.

5. A 16-year-old woman collapses at home. She had been arguing with her mother who has found out that she is on the contraceptive pill. Suddenly she appeared to have difficulty in breathing. On examination, she is tachypnoeic and is complaining of chest pain. Her lying blood pressure is 100/60 mmHg. Her arterial blood gases show a P_{CO_2} of 28 kPa and a P_{O_2} of 70 kPa.

Answers to 1.15

1. **E. Hypertrophic obstructive cardiomyopathy (HOCM).** Young fit men rarely collapse and such events should be treated seriously. Simple faints and postural hypotension are most uncommon during strenuous exertion and there is nothing in the history to suggest a pulmonary embolus (although this does not exclude the diagnosis). The finding of an ejection systolic murmur puts HOCM high on the list of differential diagnoses. Aortic stenosis would be uncommon in this age group.

2. **I. Simple faint.** Although many causes are possible, the history does not suggest a more sinister cause for the collapse. A slow pulse rate and the pale, sweaty appearance are helpful clues. Nevertheless, any further attacks would need careful assessment. *Note* that a blood pressure of 100/60 mmHg is normal in a woman of this age.

3. **G. Postural hypotension.** Light-headedness on standing should prompt exclusion of postural hypotension. Elderly patients with type 2 diabetes frequently have autonomic neuropathy. The increasingly aggressive treatment of hypertension in patients with diabetes makes postural hypotension a problem, especially if the blood pressure is only checked in the sitting or lying position in the clinic.

4. **A. Aortic stenosis.** The triad of angina, episodes of collapse and an ejection systolic murmur makes aortic stenosis the most important diagnosis to exclude. The low pulse volume further supports this as the cause of the collapse.

5. **H. Pulmonary embolus.** Care should be taken in diagnosing hyperventilation syndrome since patients with serious diseases such as pulmonary embolus or asthma may be missed. Although the history is emotionally charged, a patient with hyperventilation should not be hypoxic and complains more of dyspnoea than chest pain. The oral contraceptive pill is a risk factor for pulmonary embolus.

HEADACHE

1.16 **For each of the following patients complaining of a headache, select the most likely diagnosis.**

A   Benign paroxysmal headache
B   Cluster headache
C   De Quervain's thyroiditis
D   Essential hypertension
E   Migraine
F   Raised intracranial pressure
G   Subarachnoid haemorrhage
H   Temporal arteritis
I   Tension headache
J   Trigeminal neuralgia

1.   A 28-year-old man complains of a constant and generalized headache, which feels like a pressure on the top and a band around his head. He is unsure when it started but it has been present for at least 2 months. It is sometimes worse in the mornings but it never fully disappears, despite regular co-codamol.

2.   A 40-year-old woman complains of severe headache. She gets attacks about once a month. The headache can come on at any time, takes around 1 h to develop and lasts for the rest of the day. The headaches are often associated with nausea and photophobia.

3.   A 39-year-old woman with a history of migraine presents with a headache. She says that it is not like her previous attacks of migraine. The headache came on suddenly at the back of her head and is the worst headache she ever recalls. She has vomited with the pain, has photophobia and mild neck stiffness.

4.   A 42-year-old man complains of sudden-onset excruciating pain in the forehead and under the left eye. The pain lasts only a few seconds at a time but he has many attacks each day, mostly brought on by some activity such as shaving, chewing or washing his face.

5.   A 38-year-old woman complains of sharp severe headache at the back of her head. The attacks last around 5 min and then she feels well again. She has noticed the attacks come on after eating ice-cream or other cold foods or drinks.

Answers to 1.16

1. **I. Tension headache.** The key features that suggest tension headache include the description of a 'band around the head', long duration, failure to respond to simple analgesics, and inability to pin-point precise start and lack of pain-free periods.

2. **E. Migraine.** This is a typical history of migraine. Precipitants may include 'stress', certain foods or lack of sleep. Fortification spectra refers to the geometrical shapes that may be seen as bright lights. Some attacks may be followed by a period of hemiparesis (hemiplegic migraine). Beware of missing an intracranial vascular anomaly in a patient with recurrent migraine, especially if the symptoms are always on the same side.

3. **G. Subarachnoid haemorrhage.** A typical, full-blown subarachnoid haemorrhage is hard to miss – the patient may suddenly lose consciousness or complain of severe headache with focal neurological signs. However, the diagnosis may be easily missed in patients who present with less impressive symptoms or when they also have a history of migraine or other causes for headache. Even if initially well, 30% of patients will re-bleed and of these, at least 50% will die.

4. **J. Trigeminal neuralgia.** It is important to distinguish in the history from headache and facial pain since the list of possible causes is different. Sudden, shooting pain in the face suggests trigeminal neuralgia, and it is sometimes initiated by trivial activity involving the facial muscles.

5. **A. Benign paroxysmal headache.** Other precipitants include sexual intercourse, cough and severe exertion. The headache is usually short-lived but it may be difficult to distinguish from subarachnoid haemorrhage if of longer duration.

SEIZURES AND OTHER TRANSIENT NEUROLOGICAL SYMPTOMS

1.17 **The following patients have had a transient neurological event; select the most likely diagnosis.**

A Absence attacks
B Atonic seizures
C Complex partial seizures
D Drop attacks
E Myoclonic seizures
F Postural hypotension
G Simple partial seizures
H Stokes–Adams attack
I Tonic clonic seizures
J Vasovagal attack

1. A 23-year-old woman is out shopping and suddenly falls to the ground unconscious. Her entire body appears to go stiff and all four limbs start to jerk. The attack lasts around 3 min.

2. A 27-year-old man is noticed at work to suddenly stop in mid-conversation, staring blankly ahead. He makes rhythmic movements with his tongue as though he were licking his lips and this lasts 2 min. He then returns to normal but feels rather confused and cannot recall what he was talking about before the attack.

3. A 9-year-old boy is not progressing well at school. When he is carefully observed, it appears as though he stares blankly for around 10 s, blinking his eyelids and then returns to normal. He is not confused after these attacks, which occur several times an hour.

4. A 40-year-old man notices that his left hand and arm twitch uncontrollably for around 5 min several times a day. He is fully conscious during these attacks and tries to control them but to no avail.

5. A 13-year-old girl is waiting to pay for a CD in a local shop. She starts to feel unwell, nauseated and light-headed and slowly slumps to the ground. She is able to hold a conversation but says her vision is blurred. She returns to normal after a few minutes.

Answers to 1.17

1. **I. Tonic clonic seizures.** This is a typical *grand mal* seizure. *Note* that the term epilepsy should not be used unless the patient has had more than one attack.

2. **C. Complex partial seizures.** The seizure is complex since it involves parts of the brain dealing with awareness and is partial (or focal) because it does not involve the entire brain. These seizures last from a few seconds to a few minutes and are followed by confusion and amnesia for the ictal event, although the patient may remember an aura.

3. **A. Absence attacks.** These are a specific type of complex partial seizure also known as 'petit mal'. Unlike other types of complex partial seizure, they are usually very brief but occur frequently and are not associated with obvious post-ictal confusion. These attacks are associated with a characteristic 3/s spike and wave pattern on the EEG. These discharges begin and end abruptly without any post-ictal changes on the EEG.

4. **G. Simple partial seizures.** The attack is simple because it does not affect consciousness and is partial because it is limited to the right motor cortex.

5. **J. Vasovagal attack.** These are very common and typically occur when standing, often in crowded rooms or shops. It is important to adequately explain the nature of these attacks since they may cause great anxiety to patients and their relatives who may conclude that the cause is epilepsy or another serious neurological disorder.

DETERIORATION IN HIGHER MENTAL FUNCTION

1.18 **The following patients come to medical attention because of concerns regarding their higher mental function. Select the most likely cause in each case.**

A   Age-associated memory impairment
B   Alcoholic dementia
C   Alzheimer's disease
D   Depression
E   Frontal lobe dementia
F   HIV-associated dementia
G   Creutzfeldt–Jakob disease
H   Lewy body dementia
I   Normal pressure hydrocephalus
J   Vascular (multi-infarct) dementia

1. A 76-year-old woman is worried that she might be developing dementia. She is finding it difficult to sleep and wakes early in the morning. She has become more forgetful recently and feels she is no longer of any use to the rest of her family. A CT scan of the brain is normal.

2. The son of a 68-year-old man asks to speak to his general practitioner. He has been looking after his father since the latter had several transient ischaemic attacks and a stroke. His father has begun wandering at night, cannot dress himself and becomes aggressive when asked not to leave the house. A CT scan shows scattered areas of low density in the white matter.

3. A 27-year-old man is admitted to hospital because he says he is unable to walk. On examination, he does appear to have increased muscle tone and poor balance. He becomes progressively more withdrawn, develops myoclonic jerking and refuses any food or drink. A CT scan of the brain shows widespread areas of abnormal signal.

4. A 74-year-old man is admitted to hospital after a fall. He has a poor short-term memory. His wife says that he has become increasingly unsteady on his feet and has developed urinary incontinence. A CT scan of the brain shows a dilated ventricular system.

5. A previously shy 41-year-old man is arrested after making obscene suggestions to passers-by. His wife says that his personality has changed markedly over the last month. Physical examination reveals a grasp reflex and swelling of the optic discs.

Answers to 1.18

1. **D. Depression.** The patient has a number of features of depression including disturbed sleep, early morning waking, anxiety about health, low mood and feelings of worthlessness. Depression may mimic dementia but, in addition, some patients with early dementia develop depression.

2. **J. Vascular (multi-infarct) dementia.** The dementia is due to recurrent cerebral infarcts.

3. **G. Creutzfeldt–Jakob disease.** In this young patient, a relatively unusual form of dementia seems probable. High on the list of possibilities would be HIV, spongiform encephalopathy (e.g. Creutzfeldt–Jakob), Wilson's or Huntington's disease. The myoclonic jerks are a well-recognized feature of Creutzfeldt–Jakob.

4. **I. Normal pressure hydrocephalus.** The triad of dementia, unsteady gait and urinary incontinence should prompt this diagnosis. Insertion of a CSF shunt may lead to clinical improvement.

5. **E. Frontal lobe dementia.** Frontal lobe dementias cause early personality changes with relative sparing of the intellect. This man had a slowly growing meningioma compressing the frontal lobes.

SORE THROAT

1.19 **For each of the following clinical presentations, match the most likely diagnosis from the list.**

A Acute follicular tonsillitis
B Acute infectious mononucleosis (Epstein–Barr virus)
C Acute otitis media
D Acute viral pharyngitis
E Adenoiditis
F Chronic non-specific pharyngitis
G Diphtheria
H Fungal infection of the pharynx
I Laryngeal oedema
J Peritonsillar abscess (quinsy)

1. A 35-year-old school teacher has been seeing his general practitioner for a persistent sore throat of 2 years' duration. He has a dry cough, which is worse in the mornings. He admits to smoking 20 cigarettes a day and his stated alcohol intake is 15 pints of beer a week. He has tried various cough syrups and lozenges but his sore throat with dry cough keeps recurring after only a brief relief.

2. An 8-year-old boy is brought to his general practitioner by his mother with a sudden onset of sore throat, painful swallowing, malaise and an earache. On examination, he has a temperature of 39°C, and his tonsils are erythematous, enlarged and covered with a greyish-white exudate. His submandibular glands are enlarged and tender but auriscopy shows no abnormality.

3. A 12-year-old boy presents with a sore throat, painful swallowing and pyrexia of 3 days' duration. On examination, the tonsil, peritonsillar fossa, soft palate and the uvula are all enlarged on the right side and the uvula is pushed to the opposite side. He is febrile, drooling and his voice sounds as if he is speaking with something stuck in his throat.

4. A 14-year-old girl presents with a sore throat of 12 hours' duration. Her swallowing is painful, she has a dry, recurrent cough and she feels unwell. On examination, she is febrile (38°C), her pharynx is hyperaemic and her tonsils are congested but not enlarged.

5. A 28-year-old male nurse presents to his general practitioner with a sore throat, painful swallowing and pyrexia of 2 days' duration. He has malaise, lethargy, headache, nausea and generalized aches and pains. On examination, he is mildly jaundiced, his throat is congested with palatal petechiae, the tonsils are enlarged and covered with an exudate and he has cervical lymphadenopathy and splenomegaly.

Answers to 1.19

1.   **F. Chronic non-specific pharyngitis.** This is a common but intractable condition. Often the cause remains elusive but sinusitis, reflux oesophagitis and a pharyngeal neoplasm should all be excluded. Excessive smoking, alcohol intake, overuse of the pharyngo-laryngeal speaking apparatus and the inhalation of chalk dust in the classroom are all contributory factors.

2.   **A. Acute follicular tonsillitis.** The acute onset of the sore throat and painful swallowing, pyrexia and enlarged tonsils all point to this diagnosis. The presence of a greyish-white exudate covering the tonsils should alert the clinician to the possibility of infectious mononucleosis, agranulocytosis, acute leukaemia and diphtheria. A Paul–Bunnell test, throat swab and a differential white cell count should be carried out. The earache is the referred pain felt in the IXth cranial nerve territory (tympanic branch).

3.   **J. Peritonsillar abscess (quinsy).** This is one of the complications of acute follicular tonsillitis and develops rapidly in some untreated cases. The diagnosis is easily made on inspection. The abscess should be incised without delay under local anaesthesia.

4.   **D. Acute viral pharyngitis.** This is usually a self-limiting illness characterized by an acute onset of cough with discomfort on swallowing. There may be a systemic upset with a mild pyrexia and aches and pains. The pharynx is often congested. Throat swabs should be taken to rule out bacterial pharyngitis.

5.   **B. Acute infectious mononucleosis.** The clinical picture is a characteristic presentation of this condition with predominantly systemic involvement. The presence of icterus and splenomegaly are highly suggestive of this diagnosis. The spleen, packed with lymphocytes, is friable and tender on palpation. It is liable to rupture and should be gently and carefully palpated.

BACK PAIN

1.20 **For each of the following patients complaining of back pain, select the most likely diagnosis.**

A Arachnoiditis
B Fibromyalgia
C Lumbar spondylosis
D Myeloma
E Osteomalacia
F Paget's disease
G Prolapsed intervertebral disc
H Sacroiliitis
I Scheuermann's osteochondritis
J Spinal stenosis

1. A 17-year-old man, who regularly lifts weights at the local gym, complains of back pain that is aggravated by exercise and relieved by rest. On examination, he has a dorsal kyphosis. His bone enzymes and serum calcium are normal.

2. A 54-year-old man complains of chronic low back pain following prolonged sitting, standing or lifting at work. X-rays of the spine show expansion of the vertebral body of L4 with coarsening of the trabecular pattern. His bone enzymes and serum calcium are normal.

3. An 83-year-old man complains of low back pain. X-rays of the spine show a kyphosis but otherwise look unremarkable. The alkaline phosphatase is elevated but the other biochemical tests, including serum calcium, are normal.

4. A 64-year-old woman complains of back pain and difficulty in climbing stairs. X-rays of the lumbosacral spine are normal but Looser's zones are seen in the pubic rami. The alkaline phosphatase is raised along with the serum phosphate but the serum calcium is at the lower end of the normal range.

5. A 62-year-old man complains of sudden-onset mid-thoracic back pain. X-rays show collapse of T8 and lytic lesions in several ribs. The serum calcium is 3.2 mmol/L but the alkaline phosphatase is normal.

Answers to 1.20

1. **I. Scheuermann's osteochondritis.** This is vertebral epiphysitis of unknown aetiology seen mainly in young adult males. There may be a dorsal kyphosis. Excessive exercise, such as weightlifting, before epiphyseal fusion has occurred may be a predisposing factor.

2. **C. Lumbar spondylosis.** This is the most common diagnosis made in patients with chronic back pain.

3. **F. Paget's disease.** An isolated raised alkaline phosphatase suggests the presence of Paget's disease.

4. **E. Osteomalacia.** Bone pain and proximal muscle weakness are common symptoms in osteomalacia. The biochemical profile in this case is typical. Looser's zones are a relatively uncommon X-ray appearance and suggest advanced disease.

5. **D. Myeloma.** The bone lesions are lytic and hence the alkaline phosphatase is not raised.

LOW BACK PAIN

1.21 For each of the following clinical scenarios match the most appropriate diagnosis on the list.

A   Lumbago
B   Metastatic tumour
C   Osteochondritis
D   Osteomalacia
E   Osteoporosis and compressed vertebral fracture
F   Paget's disease
G   Post-laminectomy syndrome
H   Prolapsed intervertebral disc
I   Psychogenic back pain (abnormal sickness behaviour syndrome)
J   Spinal canal stenosis

1.   A 35-year-old labourer, while lifting a heavy sack, felt a sudden, sharp pain in his lower back. The pain radiates down the back of his thigh and calf and is associated with numbness and tingling. The straight leg raising is limited to 30° by pain on the right side, and the leg raising on the left side causes pain on the right side.

2.   A 46-year-old care assistant in a nursing home complains of an intermittent low back pain of 6 months' duration. The pain radiated down the back of her thighs but did not extend below the knees. Her general practitioner finds that she has muscular spasm over the lumbosacral region, loss of lumbar lordosis, but no neurological deficit. The straight leg raising is normal.

3.   A 52-year-old woman presents with a low back pain that comes suddenly when she has walked about 100 yards. The pain radiates down her thighs, is relieved by lying down or a short rest, but it reappears if she walks or hurries. The general practitioner finds that she walks with a stoop, all the peripheral pulses are palpable, the ankle jerks are absent and there is an ill-defined sensory loss along the lateral aspect of the legs.

4.   A 38-year-old nurse has persistent low back pain that prevents her from going back to work. Her husband is very supportive and does all the household chores. The pain is relieved by rest, increased by activity, and largely unaffected by analgesics. The straight leg raising is limited when lying but normal when sitting.

5.   A 72-year-old woman developed a severe pain in her lower back when she slipped on ice and fell on her bottom. She finds it difficult to walk because of pain. The general practitioner finds that she is tender in the region of L5. She is taking a β-blocker and a diuretic for her hypertension.

Answers to 1.21

1. **H. Prolapsed intervertebral disc (sciatica).** The pain of sciatica extends below the knee and may be associated with numbness and tingling. The straight leg raising is limited and the crossed leg pain sign is virtually pathognomonic of a prolapsed disc. The absent ankle jerk suggests the lesion at L5/S1 roots.

2. **A. Lumbago (back pain without sciatica).** The pain radiates to the buttocks but not below the knees. The absence of any neurological deficit and a normal straight leg raising confirm that there is no compression of a nerve root. Magnetic resonance imaging is the investigation of choice and often shows degeneration of disc or discs.

3. **J. Spinal canal stenosis (the cauda equina angina/syndrome).** Although the clinical picture given is characteristic of this syndrome, the differential diagnosis lies with vascular intermittent claudication. The latter is unlikely in the presence of normal pulses and can be ruled out by the cycling exercise test. The patients with the neurological angina can perform better on the cycle than when walking, while those with vascular intermittent claudication are limited on both.

4. **I. Psychogenic back pain.** Some patients develop an abnormal reaction to their sickness and acquire a subconscious liking for the benefits of their disability (the abnormal sickness behaviour syndrome). Consequently, the back pain continues unabated and tends to be refractory to analgesics. The apparent limited straight leg raising when lying but not when sitting is highly suggestive of a psychogenic lumbago.

5. **E. Osteoporosis and compressed vertebral fracture.** The sudden development of a severe pain after a minor trauma, and a localized tenderness over the L5, suggest the diagnosis which can be readily confirmed on the X-ray. The mention of the two antihypertensive drugs is a helpful hint, suggesting that the patient was not on any other drugs such as hormone replacement or calcium supplements.

PRURITUS

1.22 For the following patients complaining of itching, select the most likely diagnosis.

A   Dermatitis herpetiformis
B   Eczema
C   Lichen planus
D   Pediculosis
E   Pemphigoid
F   Polycythaemia rubra vera
G   Psoriasis
H   Scabies
I   Senile pruritus
J   Urticaria

1.   A 26-year-old housewife complains of an intensely itchy rash on the wrists. On examination, there are flat-topped, pink-purple papules with a fine white network on their surface.

2.   A 16-year-old trainee hairdresser complains of itching and soreness of both hands. On examination, there is a scaly rash on both hands with fissuring of the skin.

3.   A 68-year-old man complains of itching and soreness of both hands. On examination, the rash is mainly in the finger webs and there are associated raised, linear red lesions.

4.   A 44-year-old plumber complains of generalized itching. On examination, there are scratch marks on the skin but no other lesions. The spleen is palpable.

5.   A 38-year-old gardener complains of itching of the skin of his shoulders, arms, buttocks and knees. On examination, there are numerous excoriations and a few blisters on the extensor surfaces of his elbows and knees as well as on his shoulders and buttocks.

Answers to 1.22

1. **C. Lichen planus.** Wickham's striae is the term used to describe the characteristic fine white lines that overlie the papules in this condition. Most commonly affected sites are the wrists, shins and ankles. Pruritus may be absent. The description given is typical of this disorder, which may resolve spontaneously or respond to topical steroids.

2. **B. Eczema.** The terms eczema and dermatitis are frequently used interchangeably. Trainee hairdressers are particularly prone to problems since they spend a great deal of the day with their hands in water and in contact with shampoos, bleaches and conditioners.

3. **H. Scabies.** A rash centred around the finger webs should suggest the diagnosis of scabies. The mite *Sarcoptes scabiei* burrows into the skin, causing the linear raised lesions. The diagnosis may be confirmed by scraping the mite out of the burrow.

4. **F. Polycythaemia rubra vera.** There are several general medical conditions that may present with generalized itching, including primary biliary cirrhosis, hypothyroidism and iron deficiency anaemia. In this case, the enlarged spleen suggests polycythaemia rubra vera as the cause.

5. **A. Dermatitis herpetiformis.** Intensely itchy groups of blisters over extensor surfaces of the limbs and sometimes the back are typical of this condition. Almost all patients have villous atrophy although many do not have any symptoms of coeliac disease. The rash responds to a gluten-free diet and oral dapsone.

POLYURIA

1.23 For each of the following patients with polyuria, select the most likely diagnosis.

A   Chronic renal failure
B   Cranial diabetes insipidus
C   Diabetes mellitus
D   Hypercalcaemia
E   Hypokalaemia
F   Inappropriate secretion of ADH syndrome
G   Nephrogenic diabetes insipidus
H   Polyuric phase of acute renal failure
I   Psychogenic polydipsia
J   Urinary tract infection

1.   A 19-year-old woman attends her general practitioner complaining of a 5-day history of polyuria, dysuria and loin pain. Urine dip-stick testing shows protein ++, blood +, ketones +. Plasma urea and electrolytes are normal.

2.   A 44-year-old man is seen by the nurse at his place of work because he has been feeling tired and unwell. He has a 2-month history of polyuria and nocturia. Urine dip-stick testing shows glucose ++, ketone –, protein +. Plasma urea and electrolytes are normal.

3.   A 24-year-old man complains of polyuria and polydipsia after a head injury. His doctor suggests that he try intranasal desmopressin and he finds that this cures his symptoms.

4.   A 26-year-old doctor develops symptoms of a chest infection and decides to treat himself by taking some tetracycline that he has had at home and was returned by one of his patients. Although his chest symptoms improve, he develops polyuria, nocturia and polydipsia.

5.   A 17-year-old woman is brought to her general practitioner by her concerned mother. For the last year, she has noticed that her daughter is going to the toilet many times a day. This is especially a problem when she is out shopping and at night, when she takes several cans of soft-drink to bed with her. Urine dip-stick testing and the plasma urea and electrolytes are normal.

Answers to 1.23

1. **J. Urinary tract infection.** The history and urine findings are typical of a urinary tract infection. A mid-stream urine should be sent to the laboratory to confirm the diagnosis and for microbiological sensitivities.

2. **C. Diabetes mellitus.** This is almost certainly type 2 diabetes since there are no ketones in the urine. The proteinuria may reflect diabetic nephropathy since the patient may have had diabetes for some time before the diagnosis was made. Alternatively, it could represent a co-existing urinary tract infection, so a mid-stream urine should be sent to the laboratory.

3. **B. Cranial diabetes insipidus.** This is a recognized complication of head injuries. Response to desmopressin is confirmatory and excludes nephrogenic diabetes insipidus.

4. **G. Nephrogenic diabetes insipidus.** Out-of-date tetracyclines are toxic to the renal tubules and cause a nephrogenic diabetes insipidus.

5. **I. Psychogenic polydipsia.** The normal urine testing and biochemistry exclude many options on the list. Hypercalcaemia would be uncommon in this age group. The diagnostic choice lies between diabetes insipidus and psychogenic polydipsia. It may be difficult to distinguish the two clinically but the fact that the problem is worse when out shopping and that she drinks a lot of fluid at night suggests that excessive fluid intake is the primary cause driving the polyuria. A water deprivation test would help in the diagnosis.

KEY SYMPTOMS WITH PATHOGNOMONIC SIGNIFICANCE

1.24 Each of the following presentations contains a key symptom suggestive of a diagnosis. You are required to identify it and to match each scenario with the appropriate diagnosis.

A   Colonic obstruction
B   De Quervain's thyroiditis
C   Ischaemic colitis
D   Meningococcal meningitis
E   Peptic ulcer perforation
F   Pyonephrosis
G   Retroperitoneal sarcoma
H   Subarachnoid haemorrhage
I   Temporal arteritis
J   Upper gastrointestinal haemorrhage

1. A 28-year-old woman comes to the Accident and Emergency Unit with a headache of abrupt onset. She says that she has had headaches in the past but this one felt as if a brick fell on her head. She prefers to sit in a dark room. She is in a stable clinical state with a normal blood pressure and pulse rate.

2. A 52-year-old manual worker presents with abdominal pain and vomiting of 10 hours' duration. His pain is mainly in the lower half of the abdomen, he has vomited five times and has not moved his bowels or passed any flatus.

3. A 64-year-old woman presents with breathlessness. She says that she has been feeling unwell and her friends tell her that she looks pale. Her haemoglobin level is 8 g/dL and on direct questioning she admits that she has been passing dark tarry stools for the past month.

4. A 48-year-old builder presents with a sudden epigastric pain that spread to the flanks. He cannot get comfortable in any position. He vomited twice and the pain has been persistent for 8 h. There is guarding and tenderness in the epigastrium. His pulse rate is 110 bpm and the systolic BP is 100 mmHg.

5. A 68-year-old man with a past history of ischaemic heart disease is admitted with a sudden, severe abdominal pain. The pain started in the centre and then spread to the lower abdomen. He has been vomiting for the last 4 h and passed one motion, which contained streaks of blood. He is on digoxin for atrial fibrillation and is not taking any other drugs. The pain seems out of proportion to any signs that are minimal.

Answers to 1.24

1. **H. Subarachnoid haemorrhage – *sudden headache.*** The suddenness of a headache is a classic symptom of a vascular catastrophe. The patients often say that they felt as if something fell on or hit their head. The scenario given presents an additional key symptom of photophobia since the patient prefers to sit in the dark.

2. **A. Colonic obstruction – *absolute constipation.*** Although persistent vomiting and abdominal pain are suggestive of intestinal obstruction, this diagnosis only springs to mind because of absolute constipation. Patients with abdominal symptoms tend to be preoccupied with their bowels and usually volunteer this symptom.

3. **J. Upper gastrointestinal haemorrhage – *melaena.*** The passage of dark stools suggests upper gastrointestinal haemorrhage, usually from a peptic ulcer, but there may be more serious pathology. The patient may not take much notice of it and may present with the resultant anaemia as this patient did. An upper gastrointestinal endoscopy should be performed.

4. **E. Peptic ulcer perforation – *sudden epigastric pain.*** Although this scenario is packed with clues that suggest the diagnosis, sudden epigastric pain leading to other signs is the key symptom.

5. **C. Ischaemic colitis – *sudden central abdominal pain.*** Sudden or abrupt pain suggests a vascular event or rupture of a viscus. Here the other circumstances are suggestive of ischaemic colitis. This patient has atrial fibrillation, is not on anticoagulants, pain is out of proportion to any signs that are minimal during the initial few hours, and the passage of blood all suggest mesenteric arterial thromboembolism.

Key signs in clinical practice

PRESENTATIONS OF MALIGNANCY

2.1 For each of the malignancies listed below, select the recognized presentation from the list given.

A Acanthosis nigricans
B Autoimmune haemolytic anaemia
C Disseminated intravascular coagulation
D Eaton–Lambert syndrome
E Erythema gyratum repens
F Erythrocytosis
G Finger clubbing
H Hypoglycaemia
I Paroxysmal flushing
J Tetany

1. Medullary carcinoma of the thyroid.

2. Gastric carcinoma.

3. Renal cell carcinoma.

4. Carcinoid tumour.

5. Insulinoma.

Answers to 2.1

1. **J. Tetany.** Medullary carcinoma of the thyroid produces calcitonin and may occasionally present with hypocalcaemia and tetany.

2. **A. Acanthosis nigricans.** This has the appearance of thickened, dark folds of skin in the axillae. It is also seen in insulin resistant states.

3. **F. Erythrocytosis.** Renal cell carcinoma may produce erythropoietin.

4. **I. Paroxysmal flushing.** This symptom only occurs once the carcinoid has metastasized (to the lungs or liver).

5. **H. Hypoglycaemia.** Spontaneous fasting hypoglycaemia is a presenting feature of insulinomas. These tumours may be very small lesions in the pancreas but cause severe metabolic effects.

SWELLINGS FOUND IN THE ABDOMEN

2.2 **For each of the following patients, select the most likely diagnosis:**

A   Epigastric hernia
B   Femoral aneurysm
C   Femoral hernia
D   Hiatus hernia
E   Incisional hernia
F   Inguinal hernia
G   Obturator hernia
H   Paraumbilical hernia
I   Retractile testes
J   Undescended testis

1. A 32-year-old woman presents with a painful lump in her right groin. It is not reducible and is situated 1 inch below and lateral to the pubic tubercle. There is no palpable cough impulse.

2. A 20-year-old man presents with a lump in the right groin. It appears on standing and disappears when he lies down. On examination, in the standing position, the lump can be seen above the inguinal ligament. It is reducible and displays a cough impulse.

3. A 16-year-old boy presents with a lump in the right inguinal region. It is not reducible, feels firm and is about 3 cm in diameter. There is no cough impulse. No masses can be felt in the right side of the scrotum.

4. A 45-year-old man presents with a 2 cm lump situated midway between the xiphoid process and the umbilicus. It is occasionally painful and can be reduced with gentle pressure.

5. A 65-year-old man presents with a swelling around the umbilicus, which is painless, reducible and displays a cough impulse.

Answers to 2.2

1. **C. Femoral hernia.** A femoral hernia consists of protrusion of the peritoneum (which may contain omentum or small bowel) through the narrow femoral canal, causing pain and discomfort. It can be distinguished from the inguinal hernia, which passes above and medial to the pubic tubercle.

2. **F. Inguinal hernia.** It is the most common hernia in the groin and occurs mostly in males. They are of two types, direct and indirect. The indirect hernia enters the deep inguinal ring and passes through the inguinal canal. The direct hernia protrudes through the transversalis fascia and enters the inguinal canal through the posterior wall. Long-standing inguinal hernia, especially the indirect one, may become irreducible and strangulated.

3. **J. Undescended testis.** The testes develop within the abdomen during the intrauterine life and descend into the scrotum by the time of the birth. Sometimes the descent is arrested, most commonly in the inguinal canal. Such testes are often structurally abnormal and are at risk of malignancy, especially if they are retained in the abdomen. Orchidopexy (positioning of the testis within the scrotum) should be performed.

4. **A. Epigastric hernia.** An epigastric hernia occurs through the linea alba anywhere between the xiphoid process and the umbilicus, usually midway between the two structures. It starts as a protrusion of extraperitoneal fat through the linea alba, where the latter is pierced by a small blood vessel.

5. **H. Paraumbilical hernia.** Paraumbilical herniae occur around the umbilicus and are congenital in young children and acquired in adult life. The protrusion of the abdominal contents is caused by the weakness of the abdominal wall.

SIGNS OF INTERNAL INJURY

2.3 **For each of the following scenarios, select the most likely matching sign.**

A   Ballance's sign
B   Battle's sign
C   Branham's sign
D   Bur spots
E   Carnett's test
F   Cullen's sign
G   Grey Turner's sign
H   Kehr's sign
I   Murphy's sign
J   Panda sign

1. A 5-year-old boy falls on his face while climbing a tree. He quickly gets up without any apparent injury. Four days later, he presents with diplopia and bilateral black eyes. Examination reveals bilateral bluish discoloration of the orbit and one-third cranial nerve palsy on the left side.

2. A 35-year-old man is admitted after a road traffic accident. He is hypotensive and complains of abdominal pain. His abdomen is distended and shifting dullness is obtainable on the left side but the right flank is persistently dull even when the patient is turned on his right side.

3. A 35-year-old window cleaner falls off his ladder and lands on his back. He is admitted to hospital for observation. The next day, the House Officer notices a bruise over his left mastoid process.

4. A 40-year-old motorcyclist was admitted after an accident when he collided against a lorry. He sustained abdominal injuries but his pain is localized to his left shoulder.

5. A 70-year-old man was found lying on the pavement by a passer-by, who rang for an ambulance and had him admitted to hospital. In the A&E room, he said to the doctor that he had been mugged by two teenagers who had repeatedly kicked him on the abdomen. Two days later, bruising is noticed around his umbilicus.

Answers to 2.3

1. **J. Panda sign.** Orbital pigmentation, or raccoon eyes (also called panda sign), caused by the discoloration of extravasated blood, is an important sign of a fracture of the base of skull involving the anterior cranial fossa. This can be a valuable sign in an unconscious patient when no history is forthcoming.

2. **A. Ballance's sign.** Fixed dullness on the left side with shifting dullness elicitable on the right side is caused by the presence of intraperitoneal and extraperitoneal bleeding after a splenic rupture.

3. **B. Battle's sign.** Bruising over the mastoid process is caused by extravasated blood from a fracture of the base of skull involving the petrous temporal bone.

4. **H. Kehr's sign.** The referred pain in the left shoulder is caused by splenic rupture and involvement of the diaphragm. O'Connell's modification of Kehr's shoulder sign, of rupture of the spleen, is to elicit this pain when the foot of the bed is raised.

5. **F. Cullen's sign.** This is a rare but valuable sign of intra-abdominal trauma, acute haemorrhagic pancreatitis and ectopic pregnancy. The blood dissects its way anteriorly towards the umbilicus causing the discoloration of the overlying skin. A similar bruising may occur in the flanks in acute haemorrhagic pancreatitis (Grey Turner's sign).

ABNORMALITIES OF THE PULSE

2.4 **For each of the following patients, select the pulse character most likely to be found on examination.**

A   Irregularly irregular pulse
B   Large volume pulse
C   Pulsus alternans
D   Pulsus bisferiens
E   Pulsus paradoxus
F   Radio-femoral delay
G   Sinus arrhythmia
H   Sinus bradycardia
I   Sinus tachycardia
J   Small volume pulse

1. A 19-year-old man was admitted with a suspected fractured humerus after a road traffic accident. The heart sounds are normal.

2. An 82-year-old man was admitted after a collapse. The second heart sound is soft and there is an ejection systolic murmur that radiates to the neck.

3. A 48-year-old woman with a history of chronic alcohol abuse was admitted after being found unconscious. On examination, she is covered in bruises, the right pupil is dilated and she has a laceration on her scalp. The heart sounds are normal.

4. A 58-year-old man was admitted with a 1-day history of shortness of breath. On examination, the heart sounds are soft and there is a loud and early diastolic murmur along the left sternal edge, best heard in expiration.

5. A 52-year-old woman complains of sudden onset shortness of breath 3 days after an anterior myocardial infarction. Her heart sounds are soft and the chest X-ray shows a large, globular cardiac outline.

Answers to 2.4

1. **I. Sinus tachycardia.** Pain and anxiety are the most common causes of a sinus tachycardia. Beware of patients with a tachycardia and a small volume pulse as this may indicate occult blood loss, e.g. ruptured spleen.

2. **J. Small volume pulse.** The auscultatory findings suggest aortic stenosis and this diagnosis must always be considered in elderly patients who collapse and have an ejection systolic murmur. The pulse is typically slow rising and of low volume. The soft second sound is a good pointer to the diagnosis.

3. **H. Sinus bradycardia.** The history suggests significant head injury and raised intracranial pressure, perhaps from a subdural or extradural haematoma. A dilated right pupil suggests compression of the right IIIrd cranial nerve from uncal herniation. These are relatively common in patients with a history of alcohol abuse. Sinus bradycardia is an important sign of raised intracranial pressure.

4. **B. Large volume pulse.** The patient has developed acute aortic regurgitation. Possible causes include bacterial endocarditis or an aneurysm of the ascending aorta. A large volume, collapsing (water-hammer) pulse is characteristic.

5. **E. Pulsus paradoxus.** The important diagnosis to consider is pericardial tamponade due to left ventricular wall rupture following the myocardial infarct. This characteristically occurs after 3 or 4 days and is in keeping with the chest X-ray and auscultatory findings. Normally, the systolic blood pressure (and hence the pulse volume) falls a small amount during inspiration (<10 mmHg). In pericardial tamponade, the fall is greatly exaggerated (as a result of a reduced left ventricular stroke volume) so that the pulse may disappear when a patient is asked to take a deep breath in.

THE JUGULAR VENOUS PRESSURE

2.5 **For each of the following clinical scenarios, select the most likely clinical finding on examination of the vessels in the neck.**

A   Absent *a* wave
B   Absent hepato-jugular reflux
C   Cannon waves
D   Fixed raised JVP
E   Giant *v* wave
F   Kussmaul's sign
G   Pulsus paradoxus
H   Steep *x* descent
I   Steep *y* descent
J   Venous hum

1. A patient with complete heart block.

2. A patient with tricuspid regurgitation.

3. A patient with 'lone' atrial fibrillation.

4. A patient who has recently had a large gastrointestinal haemorrhage.

5. A patient with constrictive pericarditis.

Answers to 2.5

1. **C. Cannon waves.** The *a* wave in the jugular venous pressure is due to atrial contraction. In complete heart block, there is dissociation of atrial and ventricular contraction and sometimes the atrium contracts during ventricular systole, when the tricuspid valve is closed. This results in a large *a* wave, termed a cannon wave, which occurs irregularly in complete heart block. The other cause of irregular cannon waves is multiple ventricular ectopics.

2. **E. Giant *v* wave.** The *v* wave is normally a rather indistinct 'increasing fullness' of the jugular vein as it fills during ventricular systole; blood is returning to the right atrium but has nowhere else to go since the tricuspid valve is closed. In tricuspid regurgitation, during each ventricular systole, there is a large back-flow of blood to the right atrium and jugular vein, and the entire energy of right ventricular contraction is transmitted to the jugular venous system. This large wave is the giant *v* wave.

3. **A. Absent *a* wave.** The *a* wave is due to atrial contraction and is therefore absent in atrial fibrillation. Clinically this helps in distinguishing the different causes of an irregular pulse.

4. **B. Absent hepato-jugular reflux.** Even in patients without a visible jugular venous pulse, the internal jugular vein becomes visible following firm pressure on the abdomen since this pressure is transmitted into the great veins of the neck. The absence of this finding suggests hypovolaemia.

5. **I. Steep *y* descent.** The *y* descent follows the *v* wave and is due to blood entering the right ventricle as ventricular systole comes to an end and the tricuspid valve opens. It therefore precedes the *a* wave of atrial contraction. In constrictive pericarditis, blood initially rushes into the ventricle, resulting in the steep *y* descent. A steep *y* descent may also be a feature of tricuspid regurgitation, but the primary feature of the venous pressure in this case is the giant *v* wave.

HEART SOUNDS

2.6 **For each of the following cardiac abnormalities, select the most likely finding on examination of the heart.**

A   Continuous murmur
B   Diastolic thrill
C   Ejection systolic murmur loudest with expiration
D   Fixed splitting of first heart sound
E   Fixed splitting of second heart sound
F   Loud first heart sound
G   Mid-systolic click
H   Pansystolic murmur
I   Reversed splitting of second heart sound
J   Systolic thrill

1.   Mitral regurgitation developing after a myocardial infarction.

2.   Atrial septal defect.

3.   Persistent patent ductus arteriosus.

4.   Mitral valve prolapse.

5.   Left bundle branch block.

Answers to 2.6

1. **H. Pansystolic murmur.** Mitral regurgitation is relatively common in ischaemic heart disease. Although major regurgitation, e.g. due to rupture of the chordae, may result in a palpable thrill, in most cases the finding is of a systolic murmur alone.

2. **E. Fixed splitting of second heart sound.** An atrial septal defect will result in increased flow from the right ventricle into the pulmonary artery. There is often co-existing right bundle branch block. Both of these delay right ventricular emptying so the pulmonary valve shuts markedly later than the aortic valve. Normally the pulmonary valve shuts a little later than the aortic valve on inspiration only. A pulmonary ejection murmur may also be heard in patients with an atrial septal defect but this would be loudest in inspiration and not expiration as given in option C.

3. **A. Continuous murmur.** The ductus arteriosus connects the pulmonary artery with the aorta in fetal life. The connection normally closes shortly after birth. Failure of this process causes a continuous murmur since the pressure in the aorta is always higher than in the pulmonary artery through both systole and diastole (until pulmonary hypertension supervenes).

4. **G. Mid-systolic click.** Congenital anomalies or degenerative changes may make the mitral valve 'floppy'. This may result in mitral regurgitation producing a pansystolic murmur. In milder cases, the valve does not leak but bulges into the atrium during systole, resulting in a mid-systolic click.

5. **I. Reversed splitting of second heart sound.** The second heart sound is composed of elements due to closure of the aortic valve and the pulmonary valve. Normally they occur at almost the same time but, during deep inspiration, the negative intra-thoracic pressure delays right ventricular emptying and the pulmonary sound occurs slightly later than the aortic sound (normal splitting). In left bundle branch block, left ventricular emptying is delayed and the aortic component occurs later than the pulmonary sound. Other causes of reversed splitting of the second heart sound are aortic stenosis, patent ductus arteriosus, hypertrophic obstructive cardiomyopathy and severe ischaemic heart disease.

HEART MURMURS

2.7 **For each of the following scenarios, select the most likely diagnosis.**

A   Dilated cardiomyopathy
B   Ebstein's anomaly
C   Infarction of papillary muscle
D   Infective endocarditis
E   Marantic endocarditis
F   Maladie de Roger
G   Noonan's syndrome
H   Rheumatic fever
I   Russell–Silver syndrome
J   Syphilitic aortitis

1.   A 17-year-old man has a medical examination prior to joining the Armed Forces. He is found to have a loud pansystolic murmur at the left sternal edge. He is otherwise well and has no past medical history. He is apyrexial and his full blood count is normal.

2.   A 62-year-old man is admitted to hospital with a 2-month history of increasing shortness of breath and ankle swelling. On examination, he has signs of biventricular heart failure and a soft pansystolic murmur. He is apyrexial and has a normal full blood count but his MCV is raised at 105.

3.   A 91-year-old woman with carcinoma of the breast develops a new pansystolic murmur. She is frail but otherwise well with no evidence of heart failure.

4.   A 20-year-old man is admitted to hospital with severe left ventricular failure. On examination, he has signs of aortic regurgitation and right-sided pyramidal weakness. He has an intermittent pyrexia, anaemia and a raised neutrophil count.

5.   A 12-year-old boy is found to have an ejection systolic murmur, loudest on inspiration. On examination, he is short and has webbing of the neck.

Answers to 2.7

1. **F. Maladie de Roger.** This young man appears well apart from a pansystolic murmur. The most likely cause is a small ventricular septal defect causing the loud murmur. The defect is too small to cause significant haemodynamic disorders but is a risk factor for infective endocarditis.

2. **A. Dilated cardiomyopathy.** The length of the history makes congenital heart disease unlikely and there are no criteria by which to diagnose rheumatic fever or a recent infarct. Dilated cardiomyopathy may follow a viral myocarditis or may be related to toxins such as excessive alcohol intake (would explain the raised MCV).

3. **E. Marantic endocarditis.** This is the eponymous term used to describe endocarditis developing in frail patients with malignancy.

4. **D. Infective endocarditis.** Severe left ventricular failure suggests the aortic valve has been badly damaged. The right-sided pyramidal weakness is presumably due to an embolic stroke from a vegetation on the valve.

5. **G. Noonan's syndrome.** This may occur in males or females. Patients look as though they might have Turner's syndrome, with webbing of the neck and short stature. However, chromosomes are normal. The associated pulmonary stenosis results in an ejection systolic murmur.

SIGNS ON CHEST EXAMINATION

2.8 **For each of the following pulmonary abnormalities, select the most characteristic finding on physical examination.**

A   Bronchial breathing
B   Expiratory wheeze
C   Increased percussion note
D   Increased tactile vocal fremitus
E   Inspiratory crackles
F   Intercostal muscle recession
G   Stony dullness
H   Stridor
I   Trachea deviated to the left
J   Trachea deviated to the right

1. A patient with a large retrosternal goitre compressing the trachea.

2. A neonate with respiratory distress syndrome.

3. A patient with right upper lobe fibrosis due to old tuberculosis.

4. A patient with fibrosing alveolitis.

5. A patient with a large pleural effusion.

Answers to 2.8

1. **H. Stridor.** Retrosternal goitres may displace the trachea but they are usually midline and no information is given to help to decide whether the trachea would be deviated to the right or left. However, stridor is the most characteristic feature of tracheal compression.

2. **F. Intercostal muscle recession.** This is a feature of respiratory distress. Crackles may also be heard in some cases of respiratory distress syndrome but they are not as characteristic. An increased percussion note would suggest a pneumothorax that may complicate ventilation of these small infants.

3. **J. Trachea deviated to the right.** The scarred and fibrotic right upper lobe pulls the trachea towards itself.

4. **E. Inspiratory crackles.** Patients with fibrosing alveolitis typically have fine late-inspiratory crackles, initially at the bases but then spreading throughout the lung fields as the disease progresses.

5. **G. Stony dullness.** A pleural effusion will not deviate the trachea or produce crackles or wheezes. Breath sounds are diminished and the percussion note is stony dull. A reduced percussion note (but not 'stony' dullness) occurs over areas of consolidation.

EXAMINATION OF THE ABDOMEN

2.9 Match the sign in the list with the manoeuvre described in each of the following examination routines.

A Cullen's sign
B Grey Turner's sign
C Murphy's sign
D Rebound tenderness
E Retrograde peristalsis
F Shifting dullness
G The 'board-like rigidity' sign
H The cough test
I The liver flap
J The pointing sign

1. A 38-year-old plumber was admitted with a generalized abdominal pain of 12 hours' duration. It started suddenly in the upper abdomen and within 1 h had spread to the rest of the abdomen. He vomited twice and his condition rapidly deteriorated. His heart rate is 120 bpm and the BP is 100/60 mmHg. The anterior abdominal wall feels rigid with the muscular compartment appearing like a single sheet.

2. A 42-year-old farmer was admitted with a severe abdominal pain of 6 hours' duration. The pain started in the centre and spread to the flanks and he cannot rest in any position. He is afraid to cough because it hurts and catches him in the flanks.

3. A 52-year-old housewife has been admitted with an upper abdominal pain of 4 hours' duration. She has had similar pains in the past and was admitted once before. She feels nauseated and vomited once. She localizes the area of maximum pain in the right upper quadrant. She is mildly jaundiced and pyrexial with a temperature of 38°C. She is markedly tender in the right subcostal region.

4. A 35-year-old publican is admitted with a severe abdominal pain of 6 hours' duration. On examination, he is toxaemic, jaundiced and febrile (39°C). His pulse rate is 120 bpm and the BP is 90/50 mmHg. The abdomen is tender and there is a fresh bruise around his umbilicus but he is sure that he had received no injury at that site.

5. A 12-year-old boy is admitted with an abdominal pain that started a few hours ago around the umbilicus and then radiated to the right lower abdomen. During the examination as one gently pressed over the right iliac fossa he felt pain as the hand was withdrawn.

Answers to 2.9

1. **G. The 'board-like rigidity' sign.** This is a sign of generalized peritonitis, which may result from perforation of a viscus. The overlying muscles of the anterior abdominal wall contract as a protective reflex.

2. **H. The cough test.** Cough causes pain in the flanks of the abdomen if there is inflammation affecting the parietal peritoneum. If the pain is felt in the chest then the parietal pleura is involved.

3. **J. The pointing sign.** If the patient points to the site of maximum pain and this is also the area of maximum tenderness, then the underlying viscus is likely to be the site of the pathological process.

4. **A. Cullen's sign.** This is a valuable though rare sign of acute haemorrhagic pancreatitis. A collection of blood near the umbilicus results when retroperitoneal blood dissects its way towards the umbilicus, where the colour of the overlying skin depends on the age of the bruise.

5. **D. Rebound tenderness.** This is a well-recognized sign of inflammation of a viscus and should be elicited with care and gentleness.

ABDOMINAL SWELLINGS

2.10 **For each of the following patients with a palpable mass in the abdomen, select the most likely cause.**

A	Aortic aneurysm
B	Ascites
C	Enlarged bladder
D	Fibroid uterus
E	Massive hepatomegaly
F	Massive splenomegaly
G	Ovarian cyst
H	Polycystic kidneys
I	Transplanted kidney
J	Ventral hernia

1. A 50-year-old woman with Cushingoid features has a smooth mass palpable in the left iliac fossa.

2. A 56-year-old woman with palmar erythema and numerous spider naevi has a tensely distended abdomen.

3. A 30-year-old woman admitted to hospital with a suspected subarachnoid haemorrhage has swellings in both the right and left hypochondria.

4. A 79-year-old woman complains of a swelling in the centre of her abdomen that appears when she sits up and is not present when she is supine.

5. A 67-year-old woman who is a teetotaler is admitted to hospital following a large haematemesis. On examination, she is mildly icteric and has a mass in the left hypochondrium that moves with respiration.

Answers to 2.10

1. **I. Transplanted kidney.** The patient is Cushingoid because she is on steroids to reduce the risk of graft rejection. Transplanted kidneys are felt in the iliac fossa.

2. **B. Ascites.** The woman has signs of chronic liver disease and the most likely cause of this in the UK is excessive alcohol intake. The liver may be shrunken and not palpable but a tensely distended abdomen suggests the accumulation of considerable ascites. If the ascites is not too tense, the spleen may be felt due to its enlargement as a result of portal hypertension.

3. **H. Polycystic kidneys.** There is an association between polycystic kidney disease and cerebellar haemangiomas.

4. **J. Ventral hernia.** Sitting up accentuates divarication of the recti.

5. **F. Massive splenomegaly.** This patient has had an oesophageal variceal haemorrhage secondary to long-standing portal hypertension. She has primary biliary cirrhosis.

LEFT HYPOCHONDRIAL SWELLING

2.11 **For each of the following patients with a mass palpable in the left upper quadrant of the abdomen, select the most likely cause.**

A   Carcinoma of the colon
B   Carcinoma of the pancreas
C   Chronic lymphocytic leukaemia
D   Hydronephrosis
E   Infectious mononucleosis
F   Polycystic renal disease
G   Portal hypertension
H   Renal adenocarcinoma
I   Renal tuberculosis
J   Simple renal cyst

1. A 58-year-old man is being investigated for weight loss and malaise. While in hospital, it is noted that he has a pyrexia. An indistinct, non-tender swelling is palpable in the left hypochondrium. The mid-stream urine sample shows 500 white cells, no red cells and no organisms on Gram stain.

2. A 43-year-old woman complains of recurrent bouts of colicky left iliac fossa pain, often relieved by opening her bowels. She tends to become constipated but otherwise feels well and has no weight loss. Physical examination reveals a 'doughy' mass in the left upper quadrant of the abdomen that is non-tender. The mass cannot be palpated the following day. Haematological and biochemical tests are normal but an abdominal ultrasound shows a 1×2 cm lesion in the cortex of the left kidney.

3. A 22-year-old man complains of joint pains, lethargy and malaise. On examination, a firm mass can be felt in the left upper quadrant of the abdomen. It moves with respiration and is tender. A full blood count and film is reported as showing a marked lymphocytosis.

4. A 73-year-old woman is admitted to hospital in a confused state. Her daughter says that she has recently received treatment for carcinoma of the cervix. On examination, she is dehydrated and pyrexial with tenderness and fullness of both renal angles.

5. A 47-year-old woman from Egypt is admitted to hospital following an episode of melaena. On examination, she is jaundiced and has a tachycardia. A mass is just palpable below the left costal margin and is felt better with the patient lying on her right side.

Answers to 2.11

1. **I. Renal tuberculosis.** Sterile pyuria should always prompt consideration of this diagnosis. This patient has other typical features such as weight loss and pyrexia.

2. **J. Simple renal cyst.** The history in this woman suggests irritable bowel syndrome and the masses in the abdomen that come and go are often faeces. The laboratory tests are reassuring and the ultrasound findings are most likely to represent a simple renal cyst or 'incidentaloma'.

3. **E. Infectious mononucleosis.** The spleen may become considerably distended in acute infections and rupture has been reported. Chronic lymphocytic leukaemia is a disorder of a much older group of people where the spleen is enlarged but rarely tender. Subacute septicaemia such as infective endocarditis is another cause of tender splenomegaly.

4. **D. Hydronephrosis.** Invasive cervical cancer causes obstruction of the ureters, bilateral hydronephrosis and renal failure.

5. **G. Portal hypertension.** Melaena suggests an upper gastrointestinal haemorrhage, making carcinoma of the colon a less likely diagnosis. The physical findings are of an enlarged spleen and not a pancreas. Egypt has a relatively high prevalence of chronic hepatitis B infection, leading to progressive liver failure and portal hypertension.

SPLENOMEGALY

2.12 For each of the following patients with splenomegaly, select the most likely diagnosis.

Normal values: haemoglobin 11.7–18 g/dL, MCV 82–98 fl, MCHC 31.4–35 g/dL, white cell count 3.2–11 × 10^9/L, platelet count 120–400 × 10^9/L.

A   Amoebic cyst
B   Autoimmune haemolytic anaemia
C   Cardiac failure
D   Chronic myeloid leukaemia
E   Felty's syndrome
F   Haemoglobinopathy
G   Hepatic cirrhosis
H   Pernicious anaemia
I   Sarcoidosis
J   Subacute bacterial endocarditis

1. A 34-year-old Egyptian man is admitted to hospital with a large haematemesis. He denies drinking alcohol or any history of dyspepsia. On examination, he has spider naevi and the tip of his spleen is just palpable. His haemoglobin is 10.1 g/dL (normochromic and normocytic), the white cell count is 9.6 × 10^9/L and the platelet count 800 × 10^9/L.

2. A 72-year-old Welsh woman is seen by her general practitioner complaining of tiredness and shortness of breath. On examination, she is pale and the tip of her spleen is palpable. Her haemoglobin is 5.2 g/dL (MCV 102), white cell count 2.1 × 10^9/L and platelet count 100 × 10^9/L.

3. A 30-year-old Italian man is seen at a pre-surgery assessment clinic prior to a routine hernia repair. He looks fit and well but on examination the tip of his spleen is just palpable. His haemoglobin is 10.9 g/dL (MCV 70, MCHC 21), but his white cell count and platelet count are normal. Several weeks of oral iron therapy do not improve his blood count.

4. A 63-year-old Englishman is admitted with a chest infection. This is the third such infection he has had in 6 weeks. On examination, his spleen is enlarged to the umbilicus. His haemoglobin is 11 g/dL (MCV 100), white cell count 42 × 10^9/L and platelet count normal.

5. A 40-year-old Scotsman is seen in a hospital clinic complaining of several months' increasing shortness of breath. On examination of his chest he has inspiratory crackles. In addition, he has Heberden's nodes, a tender rash on his legs and his spleen is just palpable. His full blood count is normal but his serum calcium is raised.

Answers to 2.12

1. **G. Hepatic cirrhosis.** The history and full blood count suggest a large haematemesis and there are signs of chronic liver disease (spider naevi). The spleen is just palpable, compatible with portal hypertension. Chronic hepatitis B infection is relatively common in Egypt and this man is likely to have bled from oesophageal varices.

2. **H. Pernicious anaemia.** The full blood count shows a pancytopaenia and a raised MCV. Most patients adjust well to the gradually falling haemoglobin levels and are very anaemic at the time of presentation.

3. **F. Haemoglobinopathy.** Thalassaemias are seen in people from Mediterranean regions, including Italy. Heterozygous carriers are usually asymptomatic and may be picked up because a full blood count shows an iron-deficient picture (i.e. low MCV and MCHC) that fails to respond to iron therapy. The red cells are characteristically small and contain less haemoglobin but the total red cell count is increased by about 10–20%. The diagnosis can be made by haemoglobin electrophoresis or molecular biological methods. Splenomegaly occurs only in a minority of patients.

4. **D. Chronic myeloid leukaemia.** There is massive splenomegaly and a raised white cell count.

5. **I. Sarcoidosis.** The key findings here are hypercalcaemia and erythema nodosum. The hypercalcaemia probably arises from excessive activation of vitamin D in the giant cell granulomas that are typical of the condition. Shortness of breath and inspiratory crackles suggest pulmonary involvement.

PALPABLE LIVER

2.13 **For each of the following patients with a palpable liver, select the most likely diagnosis.**

A   Acute alcoholic hepatitis
B   Acute lymphocytic leukaemia
C   Amyloidosis
D   Autoimmune chronic active hepatitis
E   Budd–Chiari syndrome
F   Emphysema
G   Fatty liver
H   Infectious mononucleosis
I   Metastases
J   Sclerosing cholangitis

1. A 55-year-old man is seen in the clinic because of poor diabetic control. On examination, the liver is palpable 3 cm below the costal margin. His liver function tests show a marginally raised ALT and bilirubin and an alkaline phosphatase twice the upper limit of normal.

2. A 19-year-old woman complains of tiredness. She has hepatosplenomegaly and several enlarged lymph nodes are palpable in the neck. Her full blood count shows a lymphocytosis with 30% atypical mononuclear cells. Her liver function tests show that the ALT, alkaline phosphatase and bilirubin are elevated.

3. A 74-year-old man has a 2-year history of declining health and gradual weight loss. He admits to smoking 30 cigarettes a day and drinking 60 units of alcohol a week. A smooth, non-tender liver edge is felt just below the costal margin. His full blood count and liver function tests are normal.

4. A 42-year-old man is admitted to hospital with a 3-week history of progressive and painless jaundice. In the last 4 months, he has had intermittent diarrhoea. He has a non-tender, hard mass in the right upper quadrant of the abdomen. His full blood count shows a microcytic, hypochromic anaemia. The liver function tests confirm a cholestatic picture.

5. A 61-year-old man visits his general practitioner complaining of pins and needles in his hands and feet. He is told to reduce his alcohol intake (previously 20 units/week). His symptoms do not improve and a physical examination shows that his liver is enlarged, is non-tender and feels firm. His full blood count and liver function tests are normal.

Answers to 2.13

1. **G. Fatty liver.** Deposition of fat in the liver is common in people with poorly controlled diabetes. The condition resolves as glycaemic control improves.

2. **H. Infectious mononucleosis.** The key to the diagnosis is the finding of atypical mononuclear cells. Acute leukaemia would have shown other abnormalities in the full blood count such as anaemia or a reduced platelet count. Massive hepatomegaly is a feature of chronic rather than acute leukaemias.

3. **F. Emphysema.** The history is rather too long for a neoplastic process. The liver function tests are normal, making intrinsic liver disease unlikely (although not impossible). In fact, this man had emphysema due to his heavy smoking habit. The enlarged lungs had displaced his liver inferiorly so that it could be palpated below the costal margin.

4. **I. Metastases.** Progressive painless jaundice associated with weight loss is an ominous symptom. Although relatively young, this man had carcinoma of the colon that had metastasized to the liver.

5. **C. Amyloidosis.** Amyloid deposition is a cause of peripheral neuropathy. The alcohol intake is insufficient to make this a likely cause of liver disease and, in any case, the liver is often shrunken and not palpable in alcoholic cirrhosis (although it is palpable and tender when fatty infiltration is a prominent feature).

ASCITES

2.14 For each of the following patients with ascites, select the most likely cause.

A Budd–Chiari syndrome
B Cardiac failure
C Hepatic cirrhosis
D Hepatocellular carcinoma
E Lymphatic obstruction
F Malignancy
G Meig's syndrome
H Nephrotic syndrome
I Pancreatitis
J Spontaneous bacterial peritonitis

1. A 58-year-old woman is admitted to hospital complaining of shortness of breath and swelling of her legs and abdomen. On examination, she has an elevated jugular venous pressure, bilateral pitting oedema to the thighs, an enlarged tender liver and moderate ascites. Urine dip-stick testing reveals glucose ++ and a trace of protein.

2. A 55-year-old woman is admitted to hospital with weight loss and abdominal swelling. On examination, she has a little ankle swelling, no hepatosplenomegaly but ascites and a right-sided pleural effusion. An ultrasound is reported as showing a mass to the left of the uterus. Urine dip-stick testing is normal.

3. A 46-year-old woman with known chronic liver disease is admitted in a confused state. On examination, she has signs of hepatic encephalopathy and tense ascites. An ascitic tap is performed. The fluid appears cloudy, the neutrophil count is 800/mm^2 and the fluid amylase 50 IU.

4. A 38-year-old woman, who is known to drink alcohol to excess, is admitted to hospital complaining of abdominal pain. On examination, she has no organomegaly but tense and tender ascites. An ascitic tap is performed. The fluid appears a little turbid, the neutrophil count is 400/mm^2 and the fluid amylase is 1500 IU.

5. A 47-year-old man with known chronic liver disease is admitted to hospital with abdominal pain and weight loss. On examination, the tip of the liver and spleen can be palpated and there is moderate ascites. An ascitic tap is performed. The fluid appears clear and straw-coloured, the neutrophil count is 5/mm^2, fluid amylase 30, but the α-fetoprotein level is markedly elevated.

Answers to 2.14

1. **B. Cardiac failure.** The most common cause of people being admitted to hospital with an elevated jugular venous pressure and ascites is heart failure. This woman also has diabetes. Other causes may need to be excluded, especially if the history is unusual or an echocardiogram shows persevered cardiac function.

2. **G. Meig's syndrome.** This is the eponymous term applied to a triad of ovarian fibroma or tumour, ascites and pleural effusion (which may be secondary to the ascites as a result of a diaphragmatic defect). It is usually seen in post-menopausal women. The removal of the ovarian lesion results in resolution of the ascites and pleural effusion.

3. **J. Spontaneous bacterial peritonitis.** The ascitic fluid has a raised neutrophil count. This is a cause of decompensation in chronic liver disease.

4. **I. Pancreatitis.** The ascitic fluid amylase is greatly elevated and the patient has abdominal pain and tenderness.

5. **D. Hepatocellular carcinoma.** α-fetoprotein is a marker for hepatocellular carcinoma. This malignancy may develop in patients with cirrhosis.

JAUNDICE

2.15 **For each of the following patients with jaundice, select the most likely cause.**

Normal values: bilirubin <17 mmol/L, ALT 5–35 IU, alkaline phosphatase 30–300 IU.

A   Alcoholic liver disease
B   Carcinoma of the pancreas
C   Choledocholithiasis
D   Drug reaction
E   Gilbert's syndrome
F   Haemolysis
G   Hepatitis A
H   Hepatitis B
I   Primary biliary cirrhosis
J   Primary sclerosing cholangitis

1.   A 73-year-old man is admitted to hospital complaining of shortness of breath. His medical history includes an aortic valve replacement and diabetes. On examination, he is pale, mildly icteric and has an ejection systolic murmur. His liver function tests are bilirubin 80 mmol/L, ALT 40 IU and alkaline phosphatase 230 IU.

2.   A 38-year-old man presents with an upper respiratory tract infection. The liver function tests are bilirubin 30 mmol/L, ALT 37 IU and alkaline phosphatase 180 IU. His medical records show that he has had a moderately elevated bilirubin level on previous occasions. He says he drinks around 10 pints of beer a week.

3.   A 64-year-old woman is referred to a hospital clinic with a 1-month history of jaundice. On examination, she is thin and admits to having lost around 5 kg in weight in the last couple of months. Her liver function tests are bilirubin 310 mmol/L, ALT 50 IU and alkaline phosphatase 1200 IU.

4.   A 40-year-old man with a history of ulcerative colitis is noted to have fluctuating jaundice. His liver function tests are bilirubin 70 mmol/L, ALT 27 IU and alkaline phosphatase 400 IU. His auto-antibody screen shows pANCA in high titre.

5.   A 61-year-old woman is seen in a hospital clinic complaining of pruritus. She complains of feeling tired and lethargic and says her only enjoyment is drinking a sherry every evening. She has bilateral xanthomata and a soft ejection systolic murmur. Her liver function tests are bilirubin 80 mmol/L, ALT 32 IU and alkaline phosphatase 440 IU. Her auto-antibody screen shows antimitochondrial antibodies in high titre.

Answers to 2.15

1. **F. Haemolysis.** The bilirubin is elevated but the other liver function tests are normal. The patient looks pale and is short of breath, suggesting anaemia. Haemolysis is occurring as blood flows across the metallic aortic valve.

2. **E. Gilbert's syndrome.** There is a history of mildly elevated bilirubin during an intercurrent illness and similar previous episodes. The alcohol intake is within medically acceptable limits.

3. **B. Carcinoma of the pancreas.** The recent weight loss is a sinister symptom in this patient with jaundice and an elevated alkaline phosphatase. There is an association between diabetes and carcinoma of the pancreas.

4. **J. Primary sclerosing cholangitis.** This is a recognized complication of ulcerative colitis. About 80% of patients are positive for myeloperoxidase anti-neutrophil cytoplasmic antibody in a perinuclear distribution (pANCA). The patient must be followed-up to exclude development of bile duct carcinoma.

5. **I. Primary biliary cirrhosis.** Pruritus is a common presenting symptom in this slowly progressive disorder that is most common in middle-aged women. Anti-mitochondrial antibodies are often found in sufferers of this disorder.

INGUINAL SWELLINGS

2.16 **For each of the following patients with an inguinal swelling, select the most likely diagnosis.**

A   Ectopic testis
B   Femoral artery aneurysm
C   Femoral hernia
D   Femoral neuroma
E   Hydrocele of the cord
F   Inguinal hernia
G   Inguinal lymphadenopathy
H   Psoas abscess
I   Saphena varix
J   Varicocele

1.   A 56-year-old man complains of a lump in the groin that he thinks might be a hernia. On examination, he has a soft, fluctuant mass lateral to the femoral artery. It does not have a cough impulse and cannot be reduced, but it can be compressed.

2.   A 58-year-old man complains of a lump in the groin. He says it gets bigger if he coughs or strains. On examination, he has an expansile and pulsatile mass below and lateral to the pubic tubercle that cannot be reduced.

3.   A 60-year-old man has noticed a swelling in the groin. On examination, there is a 4×3 cm hard and indistinct mass between the pubic tubercle and femoral artery. It is non-tender, has no cough impulse and is irreducible.

4.   A 62-year-old man presents to his general practitioner complaining of pain in his left thigh. On examination, there is a hard but smooth swelling lying lateral to the femoral artery. There is no cough impulse and it cannot be reduced. It may be moved laterally but not vertically and pressure on it reproduces the pain in the thigh.

5.   A 60-year-old man complains of a dragging sensation 'down below'. On examination, there is a swelling in the left scrotum. The testis feels normal but above it, there is a soft, compressible swelling that is limited to the scrotum. It disappears when the patient lies down.

Answers to 2.16

1. **H. Psoas abscess.** The femoral artery is an important landmark since inguinal and femoral herniae are all medial to it. The femoral vein also lies medially so the swelling cannot be a saphena varix. The femoral nerve lies laterally but neuromas are hard. This man has a 'cold abscess' from intra-abdominal TB that has tracked along the psoas sheath.

2. **B. Femoral artery aneurysm.** Pulsatility may be transmitted by any lesion adjacent to an artery; however, a swelling that is both pulsatile and expansile is an aneurysm.

3. **G. Inguinal lymphadenopathy.** It is unlikely that this swelling represents a hernia since it is irreducible and there is no cough impulse. A strangulated hernia would be expected to be tender. Enlarged lymph nodes in the groin, especially due to malignancy, commonly become matted together to form a relatively large, indistinct and hard mass.

4. **D. Femoral neuroma.** The femoral nerve lies lateral to the femoral artery. A neuroma may be due to previous trauma, an isolated finding, or a feature of neurofibromatosis. Typically, compression of the lesion causes pain in the distribution of the femoral nerve.

5. **J. Varicocele.** The lesion is limited to the scrotum and is therefore not a hernia. It lies above the testis and disappears when the man lies down – both features of a varicocele.

SCROTAL SWELLINGS

2.17 **For each of the following men with a scrotal swelling, select the most likely diagnosis.**

A   Epididymo-orchitis
B   Haematocele
C   Hydrocele
D   Inguino-scrotal hernia
E   Orchitis
F   Seminoma
G   Teratoma
H   Torsion of the hydatid of Morgagni
I   Torsion of the testis
J   Varicocele

1.   An army recruit is found to have a swelling in the left scrotum. He says it has been present for at least 2 years. On examination, there is a large swelling that is non-tender. It is possible to get above the swelling and it transilluminates brightly.

2.   A 37-year-old man is concerned about a scrotal swelling he has noticed over the last 6 months. On examination, there is a swelling in the right scrotum but it is not possible to get above it. The swelling is larger when the patient is upright and there is a cough impulse.

3.   A 14-year-old boy is admitted to hospital complaining of sudden onset severe central abdominal pain and pain in the scrotum. He has been previously well apart from a recent upper respiratory tract infection. On examination, the left side of the scrotum appears normal but the right side is swollen and very tender. The right testis appears to be lying high in the scrotum.

4.   A 27-year-old man is admitted to hospital complaining of severe pain in the scrotum that started when he awoke and has got steadily worse over the course of the day. He has previously been well apart from some dysuria over the last 48 h. On examination, the left side of the scrotum is red and tender. The testes and cord are very tender to palpation and the cord appears thickened.

5.   A 38-year-old man complains of a painless lump in the scrotum that has been present for around 3 months. On examination, the right testes is enlarged, hard and non-tender. A scar is noticed in the groin and the patient comments that this was from an operation to put the testes into the scrotum when he was a teenager.

Answers to 2.17

1. **C. Hydrocele.** Since it is possible to get above the swelling, it is not a hernia. It is non-tender, making torsion or orchitis very unlikely. Unlike a solid testicular tumour or a varicocele, a hydrocele transilluminates brightly.

2. **D. Inguino-scrotal hernia.** Inability to get above a scrotal swelling suggests it is coming from the abdominal cavity. The swelling has a cough impulse and is larger on standing, both features of a hernia, although also seen with a varicocele.

3. **I. Torsion of the testis.** Torsion is an acutely painful condition; pain may be referred to T10 because the nerve supply to the testis is derived from its original embryological position in the abdomen. The differential diagnosis includes epididymitis and torsion of the hydatid of Morgagni but in neither of these conditions does the testis lie high in the scrotum.

4. **A. Epididymo-orchitis.** The recent history suggestive of a urinary tract infection is common in this condition. Torsion of the testes or the hydatid of Morgagni are possible causes of this man's symptoms but both are rarer than epididymo-orchitis at this age.

5. **F. Seminoma.** Testicular tumours are associated with undescended and maldescended testes. Seminoma is more common than teratoma in patients over the age of 30 years.

LUMPS IN THE SCROTUM

2.18 **For each of the following patients complaining of a lump in the groin, select the most likely diagnosis.**

A Femoral hernia
B Hydrocele
C Inguinal hernia
D Sarcoma
E Seminoma
F Spermatocele
G Teratoma
H Torsion of the hydatid of Morgagni
I Torsion of the testis
J Varicocele

1. A 16-year-old boy presents with severe pain in the groin. On examination, the left side of the scrotum is swollen, tense and very tender.

2. An 18-year-old man is worried about a swelling he has noticed in his groin. It has been present for at least several months. On examination, there is a non-tender swelling in the right scrotum that transilluminates brightly.

3. A 32-year-old man complains of a swelling in his groin. On examination, there is a swelling in the right scrotum. The testes can be felt separate from the swelling but it is impossible to get above the swelling.

4. A 28-year-old man complains of a painful lump in the groin. On examination, there is a tender nodule above the right testis.

5. A 35-year-old man visits his general practitioner because he has developed tender gynaecomastia. On examination, the right testis feels irregular in shape and is larger than the left.

Answers to 2.18

1. **I. Torsion of the testis.** Severe pain and swelling of the scrotum should prompt this diagnosis. The torsion must be corrected surgically as soon as possible to prevent permanent damage to the testis.

2. **B. Hydrocele.** Lumps that transilluminate are filled with clear fluid. The fluid probably drains into the scrotum from the peritoneal cavity through a vestigial connection.

3. **C. Inguinal hernia.** If it is impossible to get above a scrotal swelling, it is coming from above, i.e. the abdominal cavity.

4. **H. Torsion of the hydatid of Morgagni.** This small structure lies on the upper pole of the testis. Torsion causes acute severe pain but, unlike a torted testis, the entire hemi-scrotum is not tender and it may be possible to localize the pain to the upper pole of the testis.

5. **G. Teratoma.** This man has a testicular tumour. Teratomas are more nodular than seminomas and may secrete chorionic gonadotrophin-producing gynaecomastia.

PHYSICAL SIGNS IN THE HANDS

2.19 **For each of the following patients, select the most likely physical finding on examination of the hands.**

A   Finger clubbing
B   Heberden's nodes
C   Hypothenar eminence wasting
D   Interosseous wasting
E   Koilonychia
F   Nail pitting
G   Nail-fold infarcts
H   Palmar erythema
I   Splinter haemorrhages
J   Thenar eminence wasting

1.   A patient with carpal tunnel syndrome.

2.   A patient with thyrotoxicosis.

3.   A patient with osteoarthrosis.

4.   A patient with bronchiectasis.

5.   A patient with psoriasis.

Answers to 2.19

1. **J. Thenar eminence wasting.** Carpal tunnel syndrome is due to entrapment of the median nerve under the flexor retinaculum at the wrist. This causes pain in the hand and forearm, sensory loss in the lateral 2$\frac{1}{2}$ fingers and wasting of the muscles that make up the thenar eminence.

2. **H. Palmar erythema.** Other causes include pregnancy and liver disease. It is also sometimes seen in normal subjects.

3. **B. Heberden's nodes.** These are bony protuberances at the distal interphalangeal joints that may be associated with deformity of the terminal phalanges.

4. **A. Finger clubbing.** Many chronic lung diseases, mostly those with an infective component such as bronchiectasis, have been associated with finger clubbing (but not asthma or chronic obstructive pulmonary disease).

5. **F. Nail pitting.** Sometimes the skin lesions are not obvious despite the presence of nail pitting. Carefully inspect sites such as the scalp, navel and natal cleft for patches of psoriasis.

ALTERED SKIN APPEARANCE

2.20 For each of the following patients, select the most characteristic physical finding on examination of the skin and mucous membranes.

A   Acanthosis nigricans
B   Central cyanosis
C   Hirsutism
D   Icterus
E   Ichthyosis
F   Pallor
G   Palmar crease pigmentation
H   Peripheral cyanosis
I   Slate grey pigmentation
J   Spider naevi

1.   A patient with severe insulin resistance.

2.   A patient with adult onset congenital adrenal hyperplasia.

3.   A patient with ectopic ACTH production.

4.   A patient taking amiodarone.

5.   A patient with Eisenmenger's syndrome.

Answers to 2.20

1. **A. Acanthosis nigricans.** This is a pigmented thickening of the skin, commonly in the axillae, back of neck and other skin flexures. It is an important clinical clue to severe insulin resistance, e.g. mutations of the insulin receptor gene.

2. **C. Hirsutism.** There is excessive male-pattern hair in a female. Usually no serious endocrine cause is found (idiopathic hirsutism). It is a feature of polycystic ovarian syndrome. In addition, milder forms of the defects in enzyme pathways that cause congenital adrenal hyperplasia in childhood may present for the first time in adult women with hirsutism.

3. **G. Palmar crease pigmentation.** ACTH and melanocyte stimulating hormone (MSH) are both cleaved from pro-opiomelanocortin and ACTH has MSH-like activity.

4. **I. Slate grey pigmentation.** Amiodarone causes numerous adverse effects including photosensitivity, corneal deposits and skin pigmentation.

5. **B. Central cyanosis.** Eisenmenger's syndrome is the term used when a left-to-right cardiac shunt (e.g. a ventricular septal defect, atrial septal defect, patent ductus arteriosus) reverses so that deoxygenated blood from the right side of the heart flows directly to the left. This is due to the development of pulmonary hypertension. Patients will also have peripheral cyanosis but this is secondary to the central cyanosis.

INVOLUNTARY MOVEMENTS

2.21 **For each of the following patients with an involuntary movement, select the most likely diagnosis.**

A   Asterixis
B   Athetosis
C   Cerebellar tremor
D   Chorea
E   Dystonia
F   Essential tremor
G   Exaggerated physiological tremor
H   Multiple sclerosis
I   Parkinson's disease
J   Wilson's disease

1.   A 36-year-old woman with thyrotoxicosis.

2.   A 57-year-old man with bronchial carcinoma finds difficulty in standing and walking. He has ataxia with his eyes open.

3.   A 37-year-old woman with an intention tremor, nystagmus and urinary incontinence.

4.   A 20-year-old woman with abrupt, uncontrolled, jerky involuntary movements and a skin rash.

5.   A 40-year-old man with a tremor of his hands that gets worse when he feels under stress and is improved by drinking alcohol.

Answers to 2.21

1. **G. Exaggerated physiological tremor.** Smoking, stress and excess thyroxine or adrenergic stimuli cause an exaggeration of the normal physiological tremor.

2. **C. Cerebellar tremor.** One of the non-neoplastic manifestations of malignancy is cerebellar degeneration.

3. **H. Multiple sclerosis.** The patient has neurological deficits in multiple sites.

4. **D. Chorea.** This woman has rheumatic fever. The rash is erythema marginatum and she has Sydenham's chorea (St Vitus' dance). The choreic movements in this disorder are usually generalized and flow from site to site unpredictably and the patient has difficulty in sitting quietly.

5. **F. Essential tremor.** There is often a family history (autosomal dominant) and characteristically the tremor is improved by drinking alcohol and aggravated by stress and writing. It may begin before the age of 25 years and persist throughout life, often increasing in intensity and spreading to other parts of the body (e.g. head).

CLINICAL SIGNS ON FUNDOSCOPY

2.22 For each of the following patients, select the most likely finding on examination of the fundus.

A   Dot and blot haemorrhages
B   Drusen
C   Flame haemorrhages
D   Hard exudates
E   Hypopigmented lesion
F   Pale discs
G   Silver wiring
H   Soft exudates
I   Spicules of pigment at periphery of fundus
J   Swollen discs

1.   A patient with chronic open angle glaucoma.

2.   A patient with retinitis pigmentosa.

3.   A patient with a melanoma.

4.   A patient with background diabetic retinopathy.

5.   A patient with a frontal lobe meningioma.

Answers to 2.22

1. **F. Pale discs.** Pale discs with increased cupping are characteristic of raised intra-ocular pressure.

2. **I. Spicules of pigment at periphery of fundus.** Early changes can be missed by indirect ophthalmoscopy since the peripheral retina may be poorly visualized.

3. **E. Hypopigmented lesion.** Although melanomas are frequently pigmented, an area of irregular pigmentation or hypopigmentation may also represent this malignant condition. Benign pigmented naevi may also occur in the fundus.

4. **A. Dot and blot haemorrhages.** *Note* that sight may be threatened by the presence of maculopathy even if the rest of the fundus just shows background changes.

5. **J. Swollen discs.** Papilloedema always suggests raised intracranial pressure. However, some patients with raised pressure never develop papilloedema so a normal fundus does not exclude the risk of coning following a lumbar puncture.

NEUROLOGICAL SIGNS IN THE EYES

2.23 **For each of the following patients with abnormalities on neurological examination of the eyes, select the most likely diagnosis.**

A   IIIrd cranial nerve palsy
B   IVth cranial nerve palsy
C   VIth cranial nerve palsy
D   Argyll–Robertson pupil
E   Holmes–Adie syndrome
F   Horner's syndrome
G   Local pupillary damage
H   Marcus Gunn pupil
I   Mitochondrial myopathy
J   Myasthenia gravis

1.   A 70-year-old woman with absent limb reflexes is found to have a dilated right pupil that fails to react to light.

2.   A 68-year-old man has a small, irregular pupil that reacts to accommodation but not to light.

3.   A 71-year-old woman has an irregularly-shaped pupil with synechiae.

4.   A 45-year-old man with long-standing diabetes complains of diplopia. On examination, the left eye looks down and out but the pupil reacts normally to light and accommodation.

5.   A 62-year-old man complains of diplopia. On examination, there is failure of abduction of the left eye but the pupil is normal.

Answers to 2.23

1.   **E. Holmes–Adie syndrome.** The lesion lies in the ciliary ganglion. Most cases are idiopathic and the condition is usually chronic and symptomless.

2.   **D. Argyll–Robertson pupil.** The lesion lies in the dorsal mid-brain. This is the classic pupillary abnormality of syphilis.

3.   **G. Local pupillary damage.** Synechiae are a sign of local disease.

4.   **A. IIIrd cranial nerve palsy.** There is failure of adduction and elevation of the eye. The cause is likely to be infarction of the nerve in this patient with diabetes. Since the parasympathetic fibres run on the outside of the nerve, they are spared and hence the pupil is normal. Pressure on the nerve, e.g. from a posterior communicating artery aneurysm, causes a complete IIIrd nerve palsy with a dilated pupil.

5.   **C. VIth cranial nerve palsy.** This supplies the lateral rectus muscle.

LUMPS IN THE NECK

2.24 **For each of the following patients with a palpable mass in the neck, select the most likely cause.**

A   Carotid body tumour
B   Cystic hygroma
C   Dermoid cyst
D   Goitre
E   Lymphadenopathy
F   Parotitis
G   Salivary gland stone
H   Salivary gland tumour
I   Thyroglossal cyst
J   Torticollis

1.   A 12-year-old girl is taken to her general practitioner because the parents are worried that she has a lump in the neck. On examination, the child appears well but has a hoarse voice due to a recent upper respiratory tract infection. Several tender lumps can be felt in the posterior triangle of the neck.

2.   At a routine 6-week check-up, a baby is noted to have a lump at the base of the neck. The parents comment that they have noted a swelling in the neck before but that it comes and goes. The swelling transilluminates.

3.   A 56-year-old woman presents with a lump in the neck. It has been growing slowly over at least 12 months. On examination, there is a 2×3 cm lump in the anterior triangle of the neck along the border of sternocleidomastoid. It is pulsatile and has a bruit on auscultation.

4.   A 10-year-old boy is noted to have a tender swelling in the midline of the neck. The parents say it has been present for a long time but seems to have become inflamed in the last few days. On examination, the swelling moves up the neck when the child protrudes his tongue.

5.   An 8-year-old girl is sent home from school because she feels generally unwell and says that swallowing is painful. That afternoon the parents call the general practice to seek advice because she has developed bilateral swellings just below and in front of her ears.

Answers to 2.24

1. **E. Lymphadenopathy.** Multiple tender lumps in the neck following a recent infection are likely to be lymph nodes. The parents had noticed only the one that was most prominent.

2. **B. Cystic hygroma.** This is also sometimes called a lymphangioma and occurs as a result of sequestration or obstruction of developing lymph vessels. The most common sites of occurrence are the posterior triangle of the neck, axilla, groin and mediastinum. This lesion typically 'comes and goes' and transilluminates brilliantly.

3. **A. Carotid body tumour.** These lesions often grow slowly and are almost always benign. The tumour arises from the chemoreceptor cells of the carotid body and transmits the pulsations of the carotid artery. The tumour may be vascular enough to have a bruit.

4. **I. Thyroglossal cyst.** Important features in the description are that the lesion is in the midline, usually below the hyoid bone or at the level of the thyroid cartilage and moves up when the tongue is protruded. There is often a history of recurrent inflammation.

5. **F. Parotitis.** This young girl with systemic symptoms and bilateral parotid enlargement has developed mumps.

LYMPHADENOPATHY

2.25 **For each of the following patients with lymphadenopathy, select the most likely diagnosis.**

A   Brucellosis
B   Epstein–Barr virus infection
C   Histoplasmosis
D   HIV infection
E   Hodgkin's lymphoma
F   Metastases
G   Non-Hodgkin's lymphoma
H   Streptococcal infection
I   Tuberculosis
J   Toxoplasmosis

1.   A 15-year-old boy presents with a sore throat, coryzal symptoms and a few tender inguinal lymph nodes. He improves spontaneously after around 10 days but returns to his general practitioner several weeks later feeling tired and lethargic. At that time, physical examination is normal.

2.   A 19-year-old woman presents with a non-tender enlarged lymph node in the neck. A biopsy shows caseating granulomas.

3.   A 16-year-old woman presents with non-tender cervical lymphadenopathy. A biopsy shows T-cells, plasma cells, eosinophils and fibrosis with a few Reed–Sternberg cells.

4.   A 30-year-old man is found to have cervical lymphadenopathy. He says the lumps have been present for over a year and do not trouble him. He is reticent to have further investigations but agrees to some blood tests. He is found to have a lymphocytosis and atypical mononuclear cells. When he returns for his results, he comments on declining vision in his left eye.

5.   A 30-year-old vet has been feeling unwell for 6 months with fatigue, a low grade fever and lymphadenopathy. He assumes he has chronic fatigue syndrome or 'ME'. However, he is admitted to hospital with a high fever and examination shows him to have a splenomegaly.

Answers to 2.25

1. **B. Epstein–Barr virus.** This is the causative agent in glandular fever or infectious mononucleosis. Patients with this condition often present with a sore throat but may also have lymphadenopathy and hepatosplenomegaly. The condition is self-limiting but persistent fatigue is not uncommonly reported.

2. **I. Tuberculosis.** Caseating granulomas are the hallmark of TB.

3. **E. Hodgkin's lymphoma.** Reed–Sternberg cells are the hallmark of Hodgkin's lymphoma.

4. **J. Toxoplasmosis.** Many infections are asymptomatic and clear spontaneously although the immunocompromised may have life-threatening disease. Active infection during pregnancy may result in congenital infection of offspring. This man was initially asymptomatic apart from lymphadenopathy. The lymphocytosis is a typical finding. Subsequently, he developed visual loss as a result of choroidoretinitis, a recognized complication of the infection.

5. **A. Brucellosis.** Farmers, vets and others in contact with farm animals may develop infection with *Brucella abortus*, although the organism is now rare in cattle herds in the UK. Subclinical infection may occur but this patient has typical features of 'undulant fever'.

LOCOMOTOR TESTS

2.26 In the following examinations, identify the test that is being carried out. Match the appropriate test with each description.

A   Heel–shin test
B   Heel–toe test
C   Rhomberg's sign
D   The abduction test
E   The Apley test
F   The Lasègue test
G   The McMurray test
H   The painful arc sign
I   Thomas' test
J   Trendelenburg test

1. A 42-year-old patient with diabetes mellitus complains in the clinic that he thinks his arches have fallen in his right foot. The clinician holds the heel of his foot in one hand, and the forefoot in the other, and then performs a see-saw motion at the ankle and twisting movements at the subtalar joints.

2. A 38-year-old patient with osteoarthrosis of his right hip walks with exaggerated abdominal lordosis. The clinician gets him to lie supine on a couch and demonstrates the lordosis by passing his hand under his spine without difficulty. He then forcibly flexes the opposite leg at the hip, which abolishes the lordosis but produces a flexion deformity in the affected leg.

3. A 14-year-old boy with a diseased right hip is walking with a limp and a tilted pelvis. The clinician asks him to stand in front of him and rest his hands, palms downwards, on his own hands held palms upwards. As the patient stands only on the affected right leg, his left hand pushes forcibly on the clinician's hand for support, and his pelvis tilts downwards on the left in an effort to regain balance.

4. A 35-year-old man with sciatica presents to a doctor who examines him on a couch. The doctor raises the man's extended leg with dorsiflexed foot without pain on the normal side, but can raise it to only 30° on the affected side. Any further upward raise was limited by pain in the back of the thigh and calf.

5. A 52-year-old man with a painful right shoulder is referred to a rheumatologist. The patient complains that he has had pain in his shoulder for over 1 week and he gets pain as he tries to lift his arm. The clinician finds that the patient experiences considerable pain as he abducts from 60° to 120°, but abduction proceeds without pain above that level.

Answers to 2.26

1. **E. The Apley test.** With the heel in one hand and the forefoot in the other, the ankle, subtalar and metatarsal mobility can be assessed. This is a useful test to check the range of movement at each joint and to localize pain.

2. **I. Thomas' test.** Flexion deformity is commonly associated with the disease of the corresponding hip. The flexion at the hip relaxes the articular capsule and lessens the pain and muscular spasm. In erect posture, this is compensated by lumbar lordosis which conceals the deformity. The presence of the flexion deformity and its relation with the lordosis can be revealed by Thomas' test.

3. **J. Trendelenburg test.** The pelvis may be tilted downwards on the non-weight-bearing side if the opposite hip is diseased, or if the abductors are weak. This can be revealed by the Trendelenburg manoeuvre.

4. **F. The Lasègue test.** This test is used to confirm irritability of sciatic nerve roots. As the straight leg is flexed fully at the hip joint, the roots of the sciatic nerve move about 2 cm through the vertebral foraminae. If the nerve is compressed or inflamed, its movement through the foramina will cause pain and will limit flexion of the straight leg.

5. **H. The painful arc sign.** The rotator cuff of the shoulder is formed by the insertions on the humeral head of infraspinatus and teres minor posteriorly, the subscapularis tendon anteriorly, and the supraspinatus tendon superiorly. Inflammation, degenerative lesions and calcium deposits in the cuff cause pain during the intermediate 60–120° of abduction, the painful arc sign.

KEY SIGNS

2.27 **Each of the descriptions given below represents a sign that has a specific relationship to a diagnosis. Match the appropriate sign with each description.**

A   Bell's phenomenon
B   Chvostek's sign
C   Confabulation
D   Cullen's sign
E   Grey–Turner's sign
F   Kussmaul's respiration
G   Murphy's sign
H   Pout reflex
I   Transillumination
J   Trousseau's sign

1.   Exert mild pressure, with the palm of your fingers, just below the right costal margin in the midclavicular line, and ask the patient to take a deep breath. As the gall bladder descends during the inspiration, it will impinge on your fingers. If it is the site of disease then this impingement will cause discomfort to the patient and he will stop in mid-inspiration.

2.   A 35-year-old publican is admitted with deep upper abdominal pain which radiates to the back. He is febrile (38°C) with a pulse rate of 120 bpm and blood pressure of 120/70 mmHg. There are signs of a left pleural effusion and upper abdominal tenderness. On the left flank of his abdomen there is a large bruise, and he denies having had any injury.

3.   Inflate the sphygmomanometer cuff round the patient's arm to a level just above his systolic blood pressure and maintain it at that level for about 5 min. The patient with hypocalcaemia may develop a painful carpal spasm, with flexion at the metacarpophalangeal joints and adduction of the thumb across the palm. The sign is positive if the spasm is relaxed about 5 s after the cuff is deflated.

4.   If a patient with a suspected VIIth nerve palsy is asked to close his eyes tightly, he is unable to close the eye on the affected side but the eyeball rolls upwards.

5.   If a lighted torch is pressed against a swelling that contains fluid, the entire swelling will light up provided the covering tissues are not too thick to allow the light to be seen.

Answers to 2.27

1.   **G. Murphy's sign.** The inflamed gall bladder (e.g. cholecystitis) will cause discomfort when it descends against the examiner's hand placed over the subcostal area below the 9th costal cartilage.

2.   **E. Grey Turner's sign.** This is a rare but reliable sign of acute haemorrhagic pancreatitis. The associated retroperitoneal haemorrhage dissects its way into the subcutaneous tissues in the flanks.

3.   **J. Trousseau's sign.** Hypocalcaemia associated with hypoparathyroidism causes a decreased threshold of excitation in nervous tissues (latent tetany), which can be detected by some simple procedures, such as Trousseau's sign. Chvostek's sign can be elicited by percussing the facial nerve just anterior to the ear lobe, or just below the zygomatic arch, where it emerges from the parotid gland. This may result in twitching at the corner of the mouth (which sometimes occurs in normal subjects), or in a more extensive contraction of the facial muscles.

4.   **A. Bell's phenomenon.** In a lower motor neurone lesion of the facial nerve, the subject is unable to completely cover the eye, and the eyeball rolls upwards in an attempt to be covered by the upper lid.

5.   **I. Transillumination.** This is a standard manoeuvre for the detection of fluid in a swelling such as a hydrocele.

EPONYMOUS SYNDROMES

2.28 **Select the most likely eponymous disorder for each of the following clinical scenarios.**

A   Berger's disease
B   Buerger's disease
C   Foster Kennedy syndrome
D   Leriche's syndrome
E   Nelson's syndrome
F   Pott's syndrome
G   Tietze's syndrome
H   Todd's palsy
I   Vincent's angina
J   Whipple's disease

1.   A 49-year-old man with coeliac disease is found to have hypertension. Further investigations show that he has impaired renal function and microscopic haematuria. A renal biopsy reveals mesangial proliferation and IgA deposits in the glomeruli.

2.   A 58-year-old heavy smoker develops rapidly progressive intermittent claudication and ischaemia of both lower limbs. On examination, no pulses can be felt below the femorals.

3.   A 51-year-old woman is admitted following a generalized seizure. She is drowsy but when she recovers complains of a 6-week history of increasing headaches and blurred vision. Fundoscopy shows that she has optic atrophy in the left eye and papilloedema in the right eye.

4.   A 74-year-old man is referred to the out-patient clinic complaining of headaches and blurred vision. His medical history includes Cushing's syndrome that was treated surgically. On examination, he is pigmented and has a bitemporal hemianopia.

5.   A 64-year-old man is being investigated for arthralgia and weight loss. His full blood count reveals him to be anaemic and an oesophago-gastro-duodenoscopy is performed. Jejunal biopsies show no villous atrophy but an increased number of macrophages in the lamina propria.

Answers to 2.28

1. **A. Berger's disease.** This is the most common form of glomerulonephritis in the UK and is associated with IgA deposits in the glomeruli. It may present with episodes of microscopic haematuria, often precipitated by intercurrent viral infections. There is an association with coeliac disease and also ankylosing spondylitis and HIV infection. This patient presented with hypertension and a raised serum creatinine concentration, poor prognostic markers. Around one-quarter of patients progress to end stage renal failure.

2. **B. Buerger's disease.** A good example of why eponymous classifications are poor, this disorder sounds like IgA nephropathy but in fact is completely different. This condition affects middle-aged smokers and there is inflammation of arteries, veins and nerves. Thrombosis in the middle-sized arteries leads to ischaemia. The precise cause is not clear but a reaction to compounds in tobacco has been suggested.

3. **C. Foster Kennedy syndrome.** A rare physical finding where a tumour on the inferior aspect of one temporal lobe causes optic atrophy on that side (as a result of ischaemia of the optic nerve) and contralateral papilloedema (due to raised intracranial pressure).

4. **E. Nelson's syndrome.** Cushing's syndrome due to a pituitary tumour producing ACTH is usually treated by a partial hypophysectomy. An alternative (now uncommonly performed) is bilateral adrenalectomy and subsequent life-long steroid replacement. Patients who have been treated with this latter approach have a risk of developing Nelson's syndrome. The ACTH-producing pituitary tumour is released from the negative-feedback control of the adrenal glands and may increase in size rapidly. The skin pigmentation is due to the stimulation of melanocytes by the excess production of pro-opiomelanocortin (the precursor of both ACTH and melanocyte stimulating hormone). The bitemporal hemianopia is due to compression of the optic chiasm by the enlarging pituitary gland.

5. **J. Whipple's disease.** This is caused by an organism called *Tropheryma whippelii*. It is a cause of malabsorption but patients often present with systemic symptoms such as arthralgia and lymphadenopathy. Jejunal biopsies show the lamina propria stuffed with macrophages containing PAS +ve glycoprotein granules. Treatment is with prolonged courses of tetracycline.

3

Cardiovascular system

SECONDARY INTERVENTION IN CORONARY ARTERY DISEASE

3.1 For each of the following interventions in patients who have had a myocardial infarction, select the approximate number of deaths avoided per 1000 patients treated per year, based on epidemiological studies.

A   0
B   1
C   2
D   3
E   4
F   5
G   10
H   13
I   15
J   18

1. Complete cessation of smoking.

2. Administration of aspirin.

3. Administration of a statin.

4. Administration of an angiotensin-converting enzyme inhibitor in a patient with heart failure.

5. Administration of a β-blocker.

Answers to 3.1

1. **I. 15 deaths avoided.** Cessation of smoking is much better for a patient than the prescription of any of the drugs listed, with the exception of the use of angiotensin-converting enzyme inhibitors in patients with established heart failure.

2. **D. 3 deaths avoided.** Studies suggest that aspirin is probably inferior to statin therapy in avoiding deaths in post-myocardial infarction subjects.

3. **E. 4 deaths avoided.** This figure is based on a reduction in total cholesterol to around 4.4 mmol/L.

4. **J. 18 deaths avoided.** Angiotensin-converting enzyme inhibitors are particularly efficacious in patients who have post-myocardial infarction heart failure.

5. **H. 13 deaths avoided.** In the past, many audit studies have suggested that β-blockers are under-used in patients after a myocardial infarction. The recent evidence that β-blockers may be beneficial in patients with heart failure has seen an increase in their use.

INTERPRETATION OF THE EXERCISE ECG (STRESS) TEST

3.2 **Match the most appropriate exercise ECG observation from the list below with the statements given.**

A   Bradycardia throughout test
B   Down-sloping ST depression (0.5 mm) including lead V5
C   Down-sloping ST depression (1.5 mm) including lead V5
D   Greater than 80% maximum heart rate reached within 5 min
E   Horizontal ST depression (1.5 mm) confined to lead II
F   Systolic blood pressure fall during exercise
G   Systolic blood pressure rise during exercise
H   Up-sloping ST depression (0.5 mm) including lead V5
I   Up-sloping ST depression (1.5 mm) including lead V5
J   Up-sloping ST depression confined to lead II (0.5 mm)

1.   The observation that generally indicates the worst prognosis.

2.   The observation that predicts coronary artery disease most strongly.

3.   The observation that predicts coronary artery disease least strongly.

4.   The observation that indicates poor fitness.

5.   The observation that indicates concomitant β-blocker treatment.

Answers to 3.2

1. **F. Fall in systolic blood pressure.** In normal individuals, systolic blood pressure rises during exercise. A fall in blood pressure is a poor prognostic indicator.

2. **C. Down-sloping ST depression of 1.5 mm including V5.** Down-sloping ST depression is a more reliable predictor of coronary artery disease than horizontal or up-sloping depression. The greater the depression, the more reliable the prediction. ST depression in the lateral chest leads has a higher predictive value than depression limited to the inferior leads.

3. **J. Up-sloping ST depression confined to lead II (0.5 mm).** Minor degrees of up-sloping ST depression limited to the inferior leads are a weak predictor of coronary artery disease.

4. **D. Greater than 80% maximum heart rate reached within 5 min of exercise.** During exercise, heart rate normally rises. Trained individuals have a lower resting heart rate and a slower rise in rate with exercise.

5. **A. Bradycardia throughout the test.** β-blockade results in a resting bradycardia and blocks the normal rise in rate with exercise. Generally, β-blockers should be discontinued prior to an exercise test.

CLASSIFICATION OF PERMANENT PACEMAKERS

3.3   **For each of the following permanent pacemakers, select the correct classification from the list below.**

A	AAI
B	AOO
C	DDD
D	IAA
E	IVV
F	VDD
G	VDDR
H	VOO
I	VVI
J	VVV

1.   A pacemaker that paces the atrium at a fixed rate with no sensing.

2.   A pacemaker that paces the ventricle. Pacing is inhibited when the pacemaker senses intrinsic ventricular electrical activity.

3.   A pacemaker that senses atrial activity and then paces the ventricle.

4.   A pacemaker that paces the atrium. Pacing is inhibited when the pacemaker senses intrinsic atrial electrical activity.

5.   A programmable dual-chamber pacemaker.

Answers to 3.3

Classification of pacemakers is based on a series of letters. The first letter of the code indicates which chamber of the heart is paced (V = ventricle, A = atrium, D = both). The second letter indicates whether the pacemaker senses intrinsic electrical activity from one or more chambers (O = no sensing, D = senses both atrial and ventricular activity, V = ventricular sensing, A = atrial sensing). The third letter indicates the response of the pacemaker to sensed electrical activity (I = inhibition, T = activation, D = dual chamber activity). An 'R' as the fourth letter indicates that the pacemaker is programmable.

1. **B. AOO**

2. **I. VVI**

3. **F. VDD**

4. **A. AAI**

5. **G. VDDR**

DISEASES OF THE MYOCARDIUM

3.4 **For each of the following scenarios, select the most likely diagnosis from the list below.**

A   Acute myocarditis
B   Arrhythmogenic right ventricular cardiomyopathy
C   Cardiac amyloidosis
D   Cardiac sarcoidosis
E   Dilated cardiomyopathy
F   Endomyocardial fibrosis
G   Giant cell myocarditis
H   Hypertrophic cardiomyopathy
I   Naxos disease
J   Restrictive cardiomyopathy

1.   A 20-year-old woman complains of poor exercise tolerance, shortness of breath and has had two blackouts. Her sister died suddenly 3 months ago. On examination, she has ankle swelling, palmoplantar keratoderma and unusual curly hair.

2.   A 56-year-old man presents with episodes of light-headedness. His general practitioner has been treating him for heart failure over the last 5 years. On examination, his pulse is 34/bpm and regular. He has a raised jugular venous pressure with visible cannon waves. A cardiac biopsy shows fibrosis and granulomas.

3.   A 23-year-old woman had pre-eclampsia during the latter part of her pregnancy. Two days after delivery her blood pressure has settled but she has worsening of her peripheral oedema and complains of shortness of breath at rest.

4.   A 17-year-old man complains of intermittent palpitations, usually after exercise. He is brought to hospital after collapsing whilst playing football. On examination, he is in sinus rhythm but has a short ejection systolic murmur at the left sternal edge.

5.   A 30-year-old woman with a history of type 1 diabetes and Addison's disease presents with severe heart failure. Her chest X-ray shows a mass in the mediastinum. A cardiac biopsy reveals a mixed inflammatory infiltrate with patchy necrosis in the myocardium.

Answers to 3.4

1. **I. Naxos disease.** This is a rare autosomal recessive disorder, mostly found in patients of Mediterranean descent, characterized by arrhythmogenic right ventricular cardiomyopathy, palmoplantar keratosis and wool-like hair. In at least some families, it is due to mutations in the plakoglobin gene.

2. **D. Cardiac sarcoidosis.** Granulomas (non-caseating) and fibrosis are typical of sarcoidosis. It may cause heart failure and damage to the conducting system may result in complete heart block (bradycardia and cannon waves in jugular venous pulse).

3. **E. Dilated cardiomyopathy.** The oedema of pre-eclampsia normally settles rapidly after delivery. Dilated cardiomyopathy may present in the post-partum period although its cause remains poorly understood.

4. **H. Hypertrophic cardiomyopathy.** Both familial and sporadic cases have been reported. In the asymmetrical form, during systole the anterior cusp of the mitral valve moves against the thickened inter-ventricular septum causing sub-aortic stenosis. Patients may present with palpitations, syncope and/or ejection systolic murmur. Some are asymptomatic and the diagnosis is only made post mortem after sudden death.

5. **G. Giant cell myocarditis.** This is an idiopathic, rare and life-threatening disease that is associated with thymomas and autoimmune disorders. Characteristically, the myocardium shows bands of necrosis surrounded by a mixed inflammatory cell infiltrate including giant cells.

PALPITATIONS

3.5   **For each of the following patients, select the most likely underlying disorder:**

A   Anxiety
B   Atrial septal defect
C   Heavy alcohol consumption
D   Heavy caffeine consumption
E   Ischaemic heart disease
F   Mitral stenosis
G   Prolapsing (billowing) mitral valve
H   Pulmonary valve stenosis
I   Thyrotoxicosis
J   Wolff–Parkinson–White syndrome

1.   A 35-year-old woman with frequent palpitations complains of sharp pains below her left breast. Auscultation reveals a mid-systolic click and a systolic murmur over the mitral area.

2.   A 70-year-old woman had sudden onset of palpitations with breathlessness 3 days ago. She is now increasingly breathless at night and needs extra pillows to feel comfortable. There is a right ventricular heave and an ejection systolic murmur over the pulmonary area. The ECG shows right bundle branch block and right axis deviation.

3.   A 45-year-old female shop assistant began to have palpitations soon after she started her new job in a soft drinks outlet. She drinks 15 units of alcohol a week, 4 cups of tea and 10 bottles of 'cola' drink a day.

4.   A 60-year-old woman has had episodes of palpitations for 6 months. She thinks she eats well but she has lost 3 kg weight in that period. Her resting pulse rate is 90 bpm and the 24-h ECG shows runs of sinus tachycardia.

5.   A 24-year-old healthy, young man has had recurrent palpitations for some months. His resting ECG shows a PR interval of 0.1 s with broad QRS complexes. A 24-h ECG shows runs of supraventricular tachycardia.

Answers to 3.5

1. **G. Prolapsing (billowing) mitral valve.** It is also called a floppy mitral valve or Barlow's syndrome. It is a common condition that is noticed incidentally on echocardiography. The mid-systolic click is caused by sudden prolapse of the mitral valve and the tensing of the chordae tendineae.

2. **B. Atrial septal defect.** The ostium secundum variety often remains asymptomatic until the onset of atrial fibrillation, which compromises left ventricular output. The right ventricular heave, systolic murmur over the pulmonary area and fixed splitting of the second heart sound are all caused by the increased flow through the right heart and right ventricular overload. In this variety, the ECG characteristically shows right axis deviation and right bundle branch block.

3. **D. Heavy caffeine consumption.** Some soft drinks such as Cola contain caffeine. The 10 bottles of this, together with 4 cups of tea a day, amounted to too much caffeine for this patient, who was unaccustomed to it until she took up this job. Caffeine, a cardiac stimulant, causes sinus tachycardia but heavy consumption may cause any arrhythmia.

4. **I. Thyrotoxicosis.** Loss of weight with a good appetite and a resting tachycardia are all suggestive of thyrotoxicosis. Although the given scenario does not mention other features of this disease, it does not match with any other condition on the list.

5. **J. Wolff–Parkinson–White syndrome.** This is a congenital condition characterized by the short-circuiting of AV conduction through an abnormal pathway. The electrical impulses conducted quickly through this short pathway produce a characteristic ECG pattern with a short PR interval and wide QRS complex. The patients get episodes of atrial fibrillation and AV re-entry tachycardia. The latter is a circus movement tachycardia in which a depolarization wave travels through the AV node and back through the abnormal pathway.

ELECTROCARDIOGRAM (ECG) ABNORMALITIES

3.6 **For each of the following 2-min rhythm-strip ECG abnormalities, select the most appropriate diagnosis.**

A   1st degree heart block
B   2nd degree heart block
C   3rd degree heart block
D   Atrial fibrillation
E   Left bundle branch block
F   Right bundle branch block
G   Supraventricular tachycardia
H   Torsade de pointes
I   Unifocal ventricular ectopics
J   Ventricular tachycardia

1. There are normal PQRS complexes, but in addition there are four QRS complexes that occur randomly but look the same as each other. They are not preceded by a *p* wave and are wider than the normal QRS.

2. There are normal PQRS complexes but the PR interval is constantly prolonged.

3. The ventricular complexes show an RsR pattern in leads V1, V2 and V3. A *p* wave precedes each complex.

4. The QRS complexes are normal in shape but the PR interval progressively increases until a *p* wave is not conducted.

5. There is a broad complex tachycardia with AV dissociation.

Answers to 3.6

1. **I. Unifocal ventricular ectopics.** Wide QRS complexes arise below the AV node or are due to abnormal conduction through the ventricle. The lack of *p* waves suggests they have originated in the ventricles. All four complexes look the same and this means the same area of the ventricle triggered the electrical discharge. They are thus unifocal ventricular ectopics.

2. **A. 1st degree heart block.** There is a delay in conduction through the AV node. Of itself, it is not associated with any specific symptoms or clinical signs.

3. **F. Right bundle branch block.** The bundle of His divides into the right and left bundles that supply the right and left ventricles, respectively. A block in conduction through the right bundle delays right ventricular depolarization so the QRS complex is widened and the leads overlying the right ventricle (V1–3) show an initial positive deflection (R), a negative deflection (s) and a further positive deflection (R), producing a characteristic 'M' shape. In right bundle branch block the initial part of the QRS complex is normal as septal depolarization, initiated from the left bundle, is unaffected. Left ventricular depolarization takes place at the normal rate but right ventricular depolarization is delayed, giving a wider QRS in the left ventricular leads and a slurred RsR pattern in the right ventricular leads.

4. **B. 2nd degree heart block.** This is also termed Wenckebach's phenomenon or Mobitz type 1 block. In Mobitz type 2, the PR interval is constantly prolonged with some *p* waves not being conducted, usually at random.

5. **J. Ventricular tachycardia.** It may be difficult to decide whether a broad complex tachycardia originates in the ventricle or is due to a supraventricular arrhythmia with a conduction defect. Lack of any association between atrial and ventricular activity (i.e. any *p* waves and the QRS) is indicative of a ventricular tachycardia.

CLASSIFICATION OF ANTI-ARRHYTHMIC DRUGS

3.7 **For each of the anti-arrhythmic drugs listed below, select the most appropriate classification.**

A Activity in all classes
B Activity in none of the classes
C Blocks AV node conduction
D Class Ia
E Class Ib
F Class Ic
G Class II
H Class III
I Class IV
J Positive inotrope

1. Amiodarone.

2. Flecainide.

3. L-sotalol.

4. D-sotalol.

5. Diltiazem.

Answers to 3.7

The Vaughan Williams classification of anti-arrhythmic drugs is as follows:

Class I: Membrane stabilizing drugs (Na^+ channel blockers)
   a. Prolong action potential
   b. Shorten action potential
   c. No effect on duration of action potential

Class II: β-blockers

Class III: Main effect is to prolong action potential

Class IV: Slow calcium channel blockers.

Thus, the correct answers are:

1.   **A. Activity in all four classes.** Although often considered a class III agent, the actions of amiodarone are complex and it has been shown to block Na^+, Ca^{2+} and adrenergic receptors.

2.   **F. Class Ic.** Flecainide.

3.   **G. Class II.** The L-isoform of sotalol is responsible for the non-cardioselective β-blocker component of activity.

4.   **H. Class III.** Prolongation of the action potential is a function of the D-isoform of sotalol. Racemix preparations (that contain equal amounts of L- and D- forms) have both class II and III activity.

5.   **I. Class IV.** Diltiazem and verapamil are slow calcium channel blockers. The nifedipine group of drugs (dihydropyridines) does not have this effect.

ADVERSE REACTIONS TO ANTI-ARRHYTHMIC DRUGS

3.8 For each of the following anti-arrhythmic agents, select the most commonly recognized adverse reaction.

A Alveolitis
B Ataxia
C Bronchospasm
D Constipation
E Flushing
F Gum hypertrophy
G Haemolytic anaemia
H Pancytopaenia
I Urinary retention
J Xanthopsia

1. Digoxin.

2. Metoprolol.

3. Amiodarone.

4. Quinidine.

5. Adenosine.

Answers to 3.8

1. **J. Xanthopsia.** A yellow-orange tinge to vision is a recognized feature of digoxin toxicity.

2. **C. Bronchospasm.** Metoprolol is more cardioselective than some other β-blockers but can still cause significant bronchospasm in patients with asthma.

3. **A. Alveolitis.** Amiodarone may produce a large range of adverse effects, including thyroid disturbance, skin pigmentation and hepatotoxicity. Among the options given, alveolitis is the most commonly recognized, leading to pulmonary fibrosis.

4. **G. Haemolytic anaemia.** Quinidine is used less often now than previously but is effective in the prevention of ventricular ectopics and atrial fibrillation.

5. **E. Flushing.** Adenosine may cause marked flushing when given by rapid intravenous injection for the treatment of supraventricular tachycardia. Bronchospasm (answer **C**) is also occasionally seen but not as commonly as flushing.

HEART FAILURE

3.9 **For each of the following patients with heart failure, select the most likely diagnosis.**

A Acute myocarditis
B Aortic stenosis
C Congestive cardiomyopathy
D Endocarditis
E Endomyocardial fibrosis
F Hypertrophic obstructive cardiomyopathy
G Ischaemic cardiomyopathy
H Pancarditis
I Pericarditis
J Pulmonary hypertension

1. A 28-year-old man presents to his general practitioner with a sore throat. He has previously been well and is reassured that no specific therapy is required. He returns 3 weeks later complaining of shortness of breath and pains in his joints. On examination, he has features of heart failure, soft systolic and diastolic murmurs, and tender, bruise-like nodules on his shins. A throat swab grows *Streptococcus viridans*.

2. A 39-year-old woman is seen in A&E after collapsing in the town centre. She recalls rushing for the bus before feeling 'faint'. She is concerned because she has had similar symptoms several times before when exerting herself and her brother has recently died suddenly of some sort of heart problem. On examination, she has a thrusting cardiac impulse, mid-systolic murmur at the left sternal edge, a 'jerky' pulse and basal inspiratory crackles.

3. A 64-year-old man with type 2 diabetes is admitted in the early hours of the morning with severe shortness of breath. He has been unable to sleep for the last week because of his symptoms, but feels a little better sitting in a chair by an open window. He also has a several months' history of increasing shortness of breath on exertion. He has been admitted on three previous occasions with acute myocardial infarctions.

4. A 43-year-old woman is admitted with a stroke. On examination, she has a dense right hemiplegia, is in sinus rhythm but has a pansystolic murmur in the mitral area, and signs of left ventricular failure. The examination also shows splenomegaly and microscopic haematuria.

5. A 30-year-old woman with systemic lupus erythematosus (SLE) develops sharp central chest pain that is worse lying back and somewhat relieved by sitting forwards.

Answers to 3.9

1.   **H. Pancarditis.** This man has post-streptococcal rheumatic fever. The rash is erythema nodosum. Rheumatic fever causes a pancarditis (endocarditis, myocarditis and pericarditis) and heart failure requiring treatment with diuretics, bed-rest and oxygen. Patients are at risk of infective endocarditis in later life.

2.   **F. Hypertrophic obstructive cardiomyopathy (HOCM).** HOCM is frequently diagnosed late since symptoms and signs may be mild until the patient has advanced disease. Although it may occur sporadically, several familial forms are recognized. Syncope on exertion, a systolic murmur and signs of left heart failure make aortic stenosis a possibility but, given the age of the patient and family history, HOCM is a more likely diagnosis.

3.   **C. Ischaemic cardiomyopathy.** This patient presents with advanced heart failure and the history of several previous infarcts makes ischaemic cardiomyopathy by far the most likely diagnosis. Controversy exists over whether people with diabetes may also have a specific 'diabetic cardiomyopathy'.

4.   **D. Endocarditis.** Septic emboli from infected cardiac valves are a common (and often fatal) complication of infective endocarditis. Microscopic haematuria is an important clue to the diagnosis, as is the splenomegaly.

5.   **I. Pericarditis.** Systemic lupus erythematosus may present with a multitude of symptoms and signs. In this case, sharp chest pain that is worse on lying is characteristic of pericarditis. Patients may also develop endocarditis and endomyocardial fibrosis, but these are not the cause of the presenting symptoms in this patient.

MANAGEMENT OF CARDIAC DISEASE

3.10 **For each of the following patients, select the most appropriate management plan.**

A   Aortic valve replacement
B   Coronary artery bypass grafting (CABG)
C   Heart transplantation
D   Heart–lung transplantation
E   Insertion of implantable defibrillator
F   Insertion of pacemaker
G   Medical treatment
H   No treatment required
I   Percutaneous transluminal coronary angioplasty (PTCA)
J   Radiofrequency catheter ablation

1.   A 79-year-old man with a history of syncope is found to have signs of moderately severe aortic stenosis.

2.   A 92-year-old woman is admitted to hospital with a history of collapse and palpitations. An ECG shows a regular rhythm but with variable PR interval and *p* wave morphology.

3.   A 24-year-old man with cystic fibrosis develops intractable right-sided heart failure.

4.   A 48-year-old man has suffered several myocardial infarctions despite previous re-vascularization procedures. He now has refractory left heart failure.

5.   A 66-year-old man with unstable angina is found to have a significant stenosis of the left main stem coronary artery. The right coronary artery has only minor atheromatous narrowing.

Answers to 3.10

1. **A. Aortic valve replacement.** The prognosis of severe aortic stenosis presenting with syncope is poor. Aortic valve replacements are performed in patients well into the eighth decade of life.

2. **F. Insertion of a pacemaker.** The ECG suggests sinoatrial disease with unstable sinus firing hence the variable PR interval and *p* wave morphology. Age is no bar to the insertion of a pacemaker and no other treatment is likely to be effective.

3. **D. Heart–lung transplantation.** Cystic fibrosis is a major indication for heart–lung transplantation. The chronic lung disease results in pulmonary hypertension and right-sided heart failure so a combined transplant is usually required.

4. **C. Heart transplantation.** The prognosis in a man of this age with severe heart failure despite full medical treatment is extremely poor. Some reports do show benefit in re-vascularization procedures (e.g. CABG) in patients with documented on-going reversal ischaemia. Otherwise, heart transplantation is the best of the options listed.

5. **B. Coronary artery bypass grafting (CABG).** A patient with a significant left main stem lesion requires urgent CABG rather than prolonged medical treatment or attempts at angioplasty.

STRUCTURAL HEART LESIONS

3.11 **For each of the following auscultatory findings, select the most likely cardiac lesion.**

A   Aortic regurgitation
B   Aortic stenosis
C   Atrial septal defect (ASD)
D   Hypertrophic obstructive cardiomyopathy (HOCM)
E   Mitral regurgitation
F   Mitral stenosis
G   Pulmonary regurgitation
H   Pulmonary stenosis
I   Tricuspid regurgitation
J   Ventricular septal defect (VSD)

1. Loud first heart sound followed by a low-pitched mid-diastolic murmur.

2. Soft second sound followed by high-pitched early diastolic murmur loudest in expiration.

3. Normal heart sounds and a high-pitched, brief early diastolic murmur loudest in inspiration.

4. Fixed splitting of the second heard sound and an ejection systolic murmur best heard in inspiration.

5. Soft second heart sound followed by an ejection systolic murmur loudest at the left sternal edge in expiration and radiating to the neck.

Answers to 3.11

1. **F. Mitral stenosis.** A mid-systolic click may precede the murmur and, if the patient is in sinus rhythm, the murmur gets louder just before the second heart sound (pre-systolic accentuation, due to atrial contraction).

2. **A. Aortic regurgitation.** This is best heard with the patient leaning forwards. Left-sided murmurs are loudest in expiration. Pulmonary regurgitation is loudest in inspiration. The aortic component of the second sound is soft because there is a lower pressure gradient between the aorta and the left ventricle at the time the valve closes.

3. **G. Pulmonary regurgitation.** A leak backwards through the pulmonary valve causes an early, high-pitched diastolic murmur. Unlike aortic regurgitation, where the murmur is loudest during expiration, this murmur is louder during inspiration because of the increased flow across the valve.

4. **C. Atrial septal defect (ASD).** There is no murmur caused by blood flowing through the defect itself. However, the increased flow through the pulmonary valve causes a flow murmur, loudest in inspiration. The delayed emptying of the right ventricle delays pulmonary valve closure so the second sound is split.

5. **B. Aortic stenosis.** *Note* that the loudness of the murmur is a poor indicator of the gradient across the aortic valve. Radiation into the neck, an associated thrill, displaced apex beat and slow-rising, low-volume pulse suggest a significant gradient. The aortic component of the second sound is soft in this case because of the reduced mobility of the calcified aortic valve.

HYPERTENSION

3.12 **For each of the following patients with hypertension, select the most likely underlying diagnosis.**

A   'White coat' hypertension
B   Acromegaly
C   Acute nephritic syndrome
D   Chronic renal failure
E   Coarctation of the aorta
F   Conn's syndrome
G   Cushing's syndrome
H   Essential hypertension
I   Phaeochromocytoma
J   Renal artery stenosis

1. A 46-year-old man is found to have a blood pressure of 170/105 mmHg each time he has it measured in the surgery. His mid-stream urine, urea and electrolytes and blood sugar are normal. On examination, his cardiac impulse is displaced and fundoscopy reveals AV nipping.

2. A 40-year-old man is found to have a blood pressure of 165/100 mmHg. His mid-stream urine and urea and electrolytes are normal but his blood sugar is 18.4 mmol/L. On examination, he has centripetal obesity, thin skin and bruising of his arms.

3. A 43-year-old woman is found to have a blood pressure of 170/105 mmHg. Her mid-stream urine shows >100 red cells, no white cells and no bacteria. The blood sugar is normal. Her urea is 23 mmol/L and creatinine 302 mmol/L. On examination, she has mild oedema of the lower limbs, her cardiac impulse is not displaced and fundoscopy is normal.

4. A 62-year-old diabetic man is found to have a blood pressure of 185/110 mmHg. His urea and electrolyte results are as follows: Na^+ 140 mmol/L, K^+ 3.6 mmol/L, urea 24 mmol/L , and creatinine 203 mmol/L. On examination, he has a displaced apex beat, absent foot pulses, bilateral carotid bruits and a left femoral bruit. He is treated with enalapril and 1 week later his urea is 48 mmol/L and creatinine 800 mmol/L.

5. A 52-year-old woman has a blood pressure of 175/100 mmHg each time it is measured in the surgery. The results of her urea and electrolytes are as follows: Na^+ 140 mmol/L, K^+ 2.8 mmol/L, urea 6 mmol/L, and creatinine 110 mmol/L. The blood sugar and mid-stream urine are normal. She responds poorly to all the antihypertensives, apart from spironolactone, which causes her blood pressure to fall to 110/80 mmHg.

Answers to 3.12

1. **H. Essential hypertension.** Over 90% of all hypertension is 'essential', in that no remediable cause can be found. There is a positive family history in almost all cases. This patient is unlikely to have 'white coat' hypertension since the blood pressure is consistently raised and there are clinical features of end-organ damage.

2. **G. Cushing's syndrome.** Hypercortisolaemia should be considered in patients with diabetes and hypertension. This man also has other features of Cushing's syndrome including centripetal obesity, thin skin and bruising. Plasma cortisol and ACTH measurements during a dexamethasone suppression test will help in confirming the diagnosis.

3. **C. Acute nephritic syndrome.** The hypertension is unlikely to be long-standing since the cardiac impulse is not displaced and fundoscopy is normal. Microscopic haematuria, hypertension and mild oedema are characteristic of the nephritic syndrome.

4. **J. Renal artery stenosis.** Deterioration in renal function may occur when patients with renal artery stenosis are given an angiotensin-converting enzyme inhibitor, such as enalapril, since this causes a further reduction in renal perfusion. Great care should be taken in prescribing these drugs to patients with evidence of significant large vessel disease (such as in this patient with diabetes and arterial bruits).

5. **F. Conn's syndrome.** Primary hyperaldosteronism, e.g. due to an adrenal adenoma, results in a hypokalaemic acidosis and hypertension. Diuretics that block the distal tubular Na/K ATPase pumps are effective in treating the condition but, if an adenoma can be demonstrated, surgery offers the best chance of long-term cure. Conn's syndrome is probably often missed since not all patients are overtly hypokalaemic. Renin and aldosterone measurements, taken in the supine position and after the patient has been upright for 4 h, help in confirming the diagnosis.

Respiratory system

BRONCHOALVEOLAR LAVAGE (BAL)

4.1   A patient undergoes bronchoalveolar lavage. For each of the diagnoses given, choose the most typical finding on analysis of the fluid.

A   0.2% eosinophils
B   1% neutrophils
C   10% basophils
D   10% neutrophils
E   40% eosinophils
F   40% lymphocytes
G   5% lymphocytes
H   60% lymphocytes
I   60% neutrophils
J   90% neutrophils

1.   A patient with pneumonia.

2.   A patient with adult respiratory distress syndrome.

3.   A patient with fibrosing alveolitis.

4.   A patient with pulmonary sarcoidosis.

5.   A patient with pulmonary eosinophilia.

Answers to 4.1

1. **I. 60% neutrophils.** In pneumonia, >50% of the cells in bronchoalveolar (BAL) fluid are typically neutrophils.

2. **J. 90% neutrophils.** Very large numbers of neutrophils are seen in the BAL of patients with ARDS. ARDS may supervene in patients with pneumonia.

3. **D. 10% neutrophils.** Patients with fibrosing alveolitis typically have a moderate increase in their BAL neutrophil count.

4. **F. 40% lymphocytes.** Pulmonary sarcoidosis is characterized by 20–50% lymphocytes in the BAL fluid.

5. **E. 40% eosinophils.** There is a variety of causes of pulmonary eosinophilia. Normally only a few (<0.3%) eosinophils appear in BAL fluid.

TUMOURS OF THE LUNG AND PLEURA

4.2 **For each of the following descriptions of intra-thoracic tumours, select the most likely histological diagnosis.**

A   Adenocarcinoma
B   Carcinoid
C   Hamartoma
D   Large cell/anaplastic carcinoma
E   Lymphoma
F   Mesothelioma
G   Metastatic adenocarcinoma
H   Metastatic melanoma
I   Small cell carcinoma
J   Squamous cell carcinoma

1.   A lung tumour that typically arises in the large airways, grows relatively slowly and metastasizes late.

2.   A tumour that arises in the periphery of the lung and is more common in non-smokers than smokers. It is sometimes associated with copious sputum production.

3.   A highly malignant lung tumour that grows rapidly and metastasizes early to the thoracic lymph nodes.

4.   A tumour that is often associated with a primary lesion in the appendix.

5.   A tumour that arises in the pleura.

Answers to 4.2

1. **J. Squamous cell carcinoma.** Since this tumour grows relatively slowly in the thorax, it may reach a large size before patients present with symptoms. Smaller, well-confined tumours that have not metastasized may be cured surgically.

2. **A. Adenocarcinoma.** These are clear-cell tumours that may produce copious amounts of mucin.

3. **D. Large cell/anaplastic.** Rapid enlargement of the thoracic nodes may lead to palsies of the phrenic nerves, invasion of the pericardium and superior vena cava obstruction.

4. **B. Carcinoid.** The appendix is a common site for primary carcinoid tumours that metastasize to the lungs and produce vasoactive peptides. Primary adenocarcinoma of the appendix is extremely rare.

5. **F. Mesothelioma.** Asbestos exposure increases the risk of both squamous cell carcinoma and mesothelioma.

RESPIRATORY MUSCLE WEAKNESS

4.3 **For each of the following scenarios, select the most likely cause of respiratory muscle weakness.**

A Botulism
B Diabetes mellitus
C Guillain–Barré syndrome
D Motor neurone disease
E Myasthenia gravis
F Organophosphate poisoning
G Periodic paralysis
H Poliomyelitis
I Shell-fish poison
J Vincristine toxicity

1. A 56-year-old man complains that when he swallows, 'the food goes down the wrong way'. On examination, he looks thin and wasted. He has fasciculation and wasting of the muscles of the hands, arms and thighs.

2. Following a suspected terrorist attack on the London underground system, several patients are taken to hospital complaining of shortness of breath and muscle weakness. On examination, they have constricted pupils, nausea, vomiting and increased sweating and salivation.

3. A 36-year-old man wakes up one morning with some cramps in his legs. When he gets out of bed, he finds both his legs are weak but he manages to struggle downstairs. He finds it difficult to hold the telephone to call for help and, by the time he is admitted to hospital, is complaining of shortness of breath.

4. A 39-year-old woman has been treated for intermittent diplopia for several years by a neurologist. However, she is now referred to the Chest Clinic with type 1 respiratory failure.

5. A 20-year-old student is found collapsed in his room. He has been vomiting and complains he is too weak to stand up. In his room, there is a large pile of tinned tuna that he has 'picked up cheap' from a friend.

Answers to 4.3

1. **D. Motor neurone disease.** There is degeneration of the motor neurones in the spinal cord and cranial nerve nuclei producing lower motor neurone signs (wasting and fasciculation). Dysphagia with nasal regurgitation of fluids and choking are common symptoms of bulbar involvement.

2. **F. Organophosphate poisoning.** Organophosphates inhibit cholinesterases in the brain and neuromuscular junction. They have been used as chemical warfare agents. Treatment is with atropine and oximes such as pralidoxime which reactivate the cholinesterase.

3. **C. Guillain–Barré syndrome.** This is characterized by a rapidly progressive muscle weakness, often ascending from lower to upper limbs and more marked proximally than distally.

4. **E. Myasthenia gravis.** The long history suggests a chronic disorder such as myasthenia gravis. Variable diplopia is a characteristic symptom of this condition. Diabetes mellitus may cause a variety of neuropathies and myopathies but rarely causes respiratory muscle failure. A IIIrd nerve palsy in diabetes may cause diplopia.

5. **A. Botulism.** This is a rare form of food poisoning caused by the toxin of *Clostridium botulinum*. Outbreaks have been associated with imperfectly tinned foods. The symptoms are of vomiting and muscle paralysis (skeletal, ocular and respiratory). In another setting, the toxin is used in cosmetic surgery (to produce 'non-surgical facelifts').

THE CHEST X-RAY

4.4 **For each of the following scenarios, select the correct radiological sign.**

A   Air bronchogram
B   Bilateral reticulo-nodular shadowing
C   Enlarged cardiac outline
D   Kerley B lines
E   Kerley A lines
F   Pulmonary nodule
G   Pleural plaques
H   Pulmonary collapse
I   Ring shadow
J   Unilateral translucency of lung field

1. Pneumonia causing distal bronchi and bronchioles to become visible as branching, linear translucencies.

2. The appearance of reduced volume in the right upper lobe and elevation of the right hemidiaphragm.

3. Hamartoma of the lung.

4. Multiple linear shadows, 1–2 mm thick and 1–2 cm long in the mid-zones and upper zones that arise from the pleura and point to the hila.

5. Poland's syndrome.

Answers to 4.4

1. **A. Air bronchogram.** Normally, the distal airways are not visible on a chest X-ray. However, in pneumonia, the lung parenchyma becomes fluid-filled and solid (consolidation) and the airways may be seen.

2. **H. Pulmonary collapse.** When looking at a chest X-ray, you should always ask yourself whether both lungs appear of equal volume. Causes of collapse include a proximal lung cancer or inhalation of a foreign body.

3. **F. Pulmonary nodule.** A hamartoma is a benign lung tumour that is sometimes diagnosed following investigation of a single nodule found incidentally on a chest X-ray.

4. **E. Kerley A lines.** These are a feature of heart failure. The more common Kerley B lines are horizontal, abut the pleura and right angles and are seen in the lower lobes.

5. **J. Unilateral translucency of lung field.** Poland's syndrome is congenital absence of the pectoralis muscle and is usually unilateral.

PATHOLOGICAL PROCESSES IN CHEST DISEASES

4.5 **For each patient below, select the most appropriate underlying pathological process.**

A   Adenocarcinoma
B   APUD cell neoplasia
C   Destruction of airways
D   Goblet cell hyperplasia
E   Laryngomalacia
F   Pleural fibrosis
G   Pulmonary fibrosis
H   Squamous cell carcinoma
I   Type 1 hypersensitivity
J   Type 3 hypersensitivity

1. A 56-year-old smoker complains of gradually increasing shortness of breath over a 5-year period. He has a cough, productive of sputum, on most days during the winter months. On examination, he has central cyanosis and signs of right-sided heart failure.

2. A 73-year-old smoker complains of gradually increasing shortness of breath over a 10-year period. He has an occasional cough. On examination, he is thin, tachypnoeic but not cyanosed. Percussion suggests he has hyperexpanded lungs.

3. A 20-year-old non-smoker complains of sudden onset shortness of breath after sterilizing some equipment at work. On examination, he is tachypnoeic but not cyanosed. Percussion suggests he has hyperexpanded lungs and auscultation reveals widespread expiratory wheeze.

4. A 59-year-old non-smoker complains of a 2-month history of weight loss (20 kg), associated with anorexia and malaise. He has developed a cough productive of large amounts of mucoid sputum. On examination, he is cachectic but there are no other abnormal physical findings.

5. A 36-year-old man complains of recurrent attacks that he describes as 'flu'. The attacks last around 3 days and consist of headache, muscle pains, shortness of breath and a dry cough. He has noticed that the attacks often occur the evening after visiting his farmer friend. On examination during an attack, he looks flushed and unwell but not cyanosed. He has fine crackles in both lung fields at the end of inspiration.

Answers to 4.5

1.   **D. Goblet cell hyperplasia.** This patient has hypersecretory chronic bronchitis and chronic obstructive pulmonary disease. Apart from hyperplasia of the mucus-producing cells, there will be loss of ciliated cells and squamous metaplasia of the respiratory epithelium.

2.   **C. Destruction of airways.** This patient has emphysema and clinically is a 'pink puffer'. The pathological hallmark is destruction of the airways distal to the terminal bronchioles (i.e. alveolar walls).

3.   **I. Type 1 hypersensitivity.** This patient is suffering an acute asthma attack. Cidex, a product used for sterilization of equipment, is a notorious allergen.

4.   **A. Adenocarcinoma.** The lack of smoking, relatively short history and sinister features in the history suggest that this man does not simply have goblet cell hyperplasia as the cause of his excessive sputum production. Adenocarcinoma occurs as commonly in non-smokers as smokers but is a relatively unusual form of lung cancer.

5.   **J. Type 3 hypersensitivity.** This man is suffering from Farmer's lung. This is a delayed hypersensitivity reaction to allergens in hay.

LUNG FUNCTION TESTS

4.6 **For each of the following, select the correct lung-function test abbreviation.**

A DLCO
B FEV$_1$
C FRC
D FVC
E KCO
F PEF
G RV
H TLC
I TLCO
J VC

1. The volume of air left in the lungs after a maximal expiration.

2. The volume of air left in the lungs after a normal expiration.

3. The volume of air exhaled in the first second of a forced expiration following a maximum inspiration.

4. The volume of air exhaled from maximum inspiration until the person can exhale no more.

5. The transfer coefficient for carbon monoxide.

Answers to 4.6

1. **G. RV.** The residual volume is the volume of air left in the lungs after maximal expiration. RV is increased in emphysema.

2. **C. FRC.** The functional residual capacity is the volume of air left in the lungs after a normal expiration. It is increased in conditions such as emphysema and asthma.

3. **B. FEV1.** The forced expiratory volume at 1s. This is decreased in chronic obstructive pulmonary disease.

4. **D. FVC.** The forced vital capacity. This is reduced in restrictive lung disorders such as fibrosing alveolitis.

5. **E. KCO.** The transfer coefficient for carbon monoxide is reduced in disorders that damage the alveolar walls where gaseous exchange occurs, e.g. emphysema.

ARTERIAL BLOOD GASSES

4.7 **For each of the following arterial blood gas results, select the most likely cause.**

Normal values: Po_2 = 12–15 kPa, Pco_2 = 4.4–6.1 kPa, pH = 7.4, [HCO_3^-] = 21–27.5 mmol/L.

A   Acute type 1 respiratory failure
B   Acute type 2 respiratory failure
C   Chronic type 1 respiratory failure
D   Chronic type 2 respiratory failure
E   Hyperventilation syndrome
F   Lactic acidosis
G   Metabolic acidosis
H   Metabolic alkalosis
I   Mitochondrial myopathy
J   Normal

1. Po_2 = 7.5, Pco_2 = 4.0, pH = 7.5, [HCO_3^-] = 24.

2. Po_2 = 9, Pco_2 = 5, pH = 7.4, [HCO_3^-] = 25.

3. Po_2 = 12, Pco_2 = 2, pH = 7.8, [HCO_3^-] = 22.

4. Po_2 = 8, Pco_2 = 8, pH = 7.2, [HCO_3^-] = 22.

5. Po_2 = 9, Pco_2 = 7, pH = 7.4, [HCO_3^-] = 32.

Answers to 4.7

1. **A. Acute type 1 respiratory failure.** The P_{O_2} is markedly reduced but the rest of the parameters are relatively normal. For example, this picture is seen in acute severe asthma. As in this case, the P_{CO_2} is sometimes a little low, resulting in a mild respiratory alkalosis.

2. **C. Chronic type 1 respiratory failure.** The patient is moderately hypoxic but all the other parameters are normal. Fibrosing alveolitis or emphysema would give this picture.

3. **E. Hyperventilation syndrome.** The P_{O_2} is normal but the patient is 'blowing off' CO_2 by hyperventilating. The P_{CO_2} is very low and this results in a raised pH. The normal $[HCO_3^-]$ excludes a metabolic alkalosis.

4. **B. Acute type 2 respiratory failure.** There is hypoxaemia but, in addition, retention of CO_2, resulting in a low pH. The normal $[HCO_3^-]$ excludes a primary metabolic cause and also suggests that the condition is acute so that metabolic compensation for the respiratory acidosis has not had time to develop. Respiratory muscle paralysis may cause this picture or an acute exacerbation of chronic obstructive pulmonary disease.

5. **D. Chronic type 2 respiratory failure.** The P_{O_2} is low and the P_{CO_2} is raised. The pH is normal due to a compensatory rise in $[HCO_3^-]$. This pattern is most often seen in patients with chronic bronchitis and chronic obstructive pulmonary disease ('blue bloaters').

CHEST X-RAY ABNORMALITIES

4.8 **Select the most likely cause for the following chest X-ray abnormalities.**

A   Aortic aneurysm
B   Dermoid cyst
C   Ectopic parathyroid
D   Foramen of Bochdalek hernia
E   Foramen of Morgagni hernia
F   Hiatus hernia
G   Lymphoma
H   Retrosternal goitre
I   Sarcoidosis
J   Thymic tumour

1.   A soft tissue mass is visible on the thoracic inlet views and is displacing the trachea.

2.   There is bilateral hilar lymphadenopathy and diffuse fibrosis in both lung fields.

3.   There is an anterior mediastinal mass on the chest X-ray of a patient with a chronic neurological condition.

4.   The mediastinum is widened on the chest X-ray of a tall, thin patient with a high-arched palate.

5.   Small intestinal shadows are visible anteriorly on a lateral chest X-ray.

Answers to 4.8

1. **H. Retrosternal goitre.** A goitre may cause significant tracheal displacement or compression with very little to feel in the neck. Thoracic inlet views are required if this is suspected.

2. **I. Sarcoidosis.** Patients with malignancy, e.g. lymphangitis carcinomatosis, may present with similar X-ray findings.

3. **J. Thymic tumour.** The chronic neurological condition is myasthenia gravis.

4. **A. Aortic aneurysm.** The patient has Marfan's syndrome. All patients with this condition require regular screening to detect widening of the aorta (by echocardiogram and/or CT scanning).

5. **E. Foramen of Morgagni hernia.** A hiatus hernia may produce stomach shadowing in the chest but not small intestine. A foramen of Bochdalek hernia lies posteriorly and is more common than the anterior Morgagni hernia.

OPACITIES ON THE CHEST X-RAY

4.9 **For each of the following patients with an opacity on their chest X-ray, select the most likely diagnosis.**

A Adenocarcinoma
B Aspergilloma
C Bronchoalveolar carcinoma
D Bronchial gland adenoma
E Carcinoid
F Hamartoma
G Haemangiosarcoma
H Metastatic carcinoma
I Non-small cell carcinoma
J Small cell carcinoma

1. A 64-year-old woman visits her general practitioner because she has lost 10 kg in weight over the last 3 months. She feels generally unwell and off her food. She has smoked 10 cigarettes a day for the last 40 years. The chest X-ray shows multiple 'cannon ball' lesions in both lung fields.

2. A 63-year-old man attends his general practice having lost 5 kg in weight over the last 2 months. On direct questioning, he admits to coughing up blood-streaked sputum occasionally over the last 2 weeks. He has smoked 20 cigarettes a day for the last 40 years. His chest X-ray shows a right hilar mass.

3. A 70-year-old man has a chest X-ray after being involved in a road traffic accident. It shows a 2 cm round nodule in the periphery of the left lung. He has smoked 20 cigarettes a day for the last 50 years. A chest X-ray performed 10 years previously shows that the lesion has not changed in that period of time.

4. A 42-year-old man is seen in the chest clinic with a 6-month history of recurrent haemoptysis. He smokes 20 cigarettes a day and has lost 2 kg in weight in the last 6 months. The chest X-ray shows an opacity in the right upper lobe with a surrounding halo of air.

5. A 58-year-old woman is admitted complaining of shortness of breath. A diagnosis of asthma was made earlier on in the year, but since that time her breathing has become worse. She has had several episodes of haemoptysis. Her chest X-ray shows several small nodules in both lung fields and prominent hilar vessels.

Answers to 4.9

1. **H. Metastatic carcinoma.** Multiple cannon ball lesions are typical of metastases. This particular patient was found to have carcinoma of the breast.

2. **I. Non-small cell carcinoma.** Blood-streaked sputum is a sinister symptom and squamous carcinoma is the most common lung cancer causing hilar enlargement in smokers.

3. **F. Hamartoma.** Previous chest X-rays can be very valuable in preventing unnecessary investigation of incidental findings on chest X-rays.

4. **B. Aspergilloma.** The halo of air is characteristic. The location, in the upper lobe, suggests that the aspergilloma has formed in an area of lung damaged by TB. However, fungus balls may occasionally develop in cavitating tumours.

5. **E. Carcinoid.** Asthma, pulmonary nodules and features of pulmonary hypertension suggest this diagnosis.

RESPIRATORY TRACT INFECTIONS

4.10 **For each of the following patients with a respiratory tract infection, select the most likely diagnosis.**

A Acute bronchiolitis
B Acute bronchitis and tracheitis
C Acute coryza
D Acute epiglottitis
E Acute laryngitis
F Acute laryngotracheobronchitis (croup)
G Atelectasis
H Bronchopneumonia
I Influenza
J Lobar pneumonia

1. A 37-year-old man develops generalized aches and pains, anorexia, blocked nose and headaches over the course of 24 h. He is pyrexial and has a cough productive of only a little sputum. Recovery occurs spontaneously after 5 days but is followed by 3 weeks of tiredness and lethargy.

2. A 36-year-old woman develops a sore throat and blocked nose with a watery discharge over the course of a few hours. After 24 h, the discharge becomes green/yellow and her voice is hoarse. She is able to continue her normal activities and the symptoms resolve spontaneously after 3 days.

3. A 19-year-old woman complains of a dry sore throat and hoarse voice that developed over a period of 24 h. She has a painful but unproductive cough and pain in her throat when she tries to speak.

4. A 5-year-old boy is brought to the general practice by his mother. He had been a little sniffly on going to bed the night before but awoke looking much worse. He has a temperature, complains that his throat hurts and is making a wheezy noise on inspiration.

5. A 6-year-old girl is taken to A&E by her mother. She says her daughter has had cold-like symptoms for a couple of days but was well enough to go to school. This morning she complained of a sore and dry throat and since then has had sudden attacks of coughing during which she looks blue. Her breathing is laboured and noisy.

Answers to 4.10

1. **I. Influenza.** Although many people claim to be suffering from 'flu', the term should be reserved for infection with one of the influenza viruses. In clinical practice, confirmation by viral culture or serology is rarely sought. Symptoms of systemic upset, joint pains and post-viral fatigue suggest that the patient is more likely to have had influenza than a common cold.

2. **C. Acute coryza.** This is the common cold. It is caused by a variety of viruses. The patient is not particularly unwell and recovers within a few days.

3. **E. Acute laryngitis.** There is no systemic upset to suggest influenza or any nasal symptoms or sputum production to suggest a lower tract infection.

4. **A. Acute epiglottitis.** Wheeze is normally heard during expiration. A wheezy noise during inspiration is probably stridor. The history is typical of acute epiglottitis. Unlike croup, there is little coughing. Attempts at visualizing the throat by asking the child to 'open wide' may result in acute obstruction of the airways by the enlarged and inflamed epiglottis and it is safer to seek urgent hospital assessment.

5. **F. Acute laryngotracheobronchitis (croup).** Croup often occurs in epidemics and follows what appears to be a minor common cold. In severe cases, there may be cyanosis and stridor, especially during the paroxysms of coughing.

ORGANISMS RESPONSIBLE FOR RESPIRATORY TRACT INFECTIONS

4.11 For each of the following patients with a respiratory tract infection, select the most likely causative organism.

A   *Actinomyces israelii*
B   *Chlamydia psittaci*
C   *Chlamydia pneumoniae*
D   *Coxiella burnetii*
E   *Haemophilus influenzae*
F   *Klebsiella pneumoniae*
G   *Legionella pneumophila*
H   *Mycoplasma pneumoniae*
I   *Staphylococcus aureus*
J   *Streptococcus pneumoniae*

1. A 22-year-old woman presents with a 2-day history of malaise, rigors, pleuritic chest pain and rusty-coloured haemoptysis. The chest X-ray shows lobar consolidation.

2. A 19-year-old woman presents with a 1-week history of headache, malaise and neck stiffness. She also complains of painful, purple lesions on her shins. The chest X-ray shows patchy consolidation.

3. A 59-year-old man who has recently returned from holiday in Spain presents with a 5-day history of malaise, dry cough, myalgia, headache and diarrhoea. The chest X-ray shows widespread shadowing in both lung fields.

4. A 42-year-old farmer presents with a 2-week history of a flu-like illness with a dry cough and conjunctivitis. On examination, he has moderate hepatomegaly. The chest X-ray shows multiple segmental opacities.

5. A 60-year-old pet-shop worker presents with a 1-month history of malaise. On examination, she has a low-grade pyrexia and hepatosplenomegaly. The chest X-ray shows patchy lower lobe consolidation.

Answers to 4.11

1. **J. *Streptococcus pneumoniae*.** This commonly affects young to middle-aged people. The 'rusty' sputum is typical as are the chest X-ray findings.

2. **H. *Mycoplasma pneumoniae*.** The purple lesions on the shins are erythema nodosum. Often there are few symptoms or signs in the chest. Meningoencephalitis is responsible for the headache, neck stiffness and confusion that may be prominent features.

3. **G. *Legionella pneumophila*.** This diagnosis is suggested by the age of the patient (often affects middle-aged and older people), the recent travel abroad (cooling towers in Spanish hotels have been the source of several outbreaks) and the gastrointestinal symptoms.

4. **D. *Coxiella burnetii*.** Farm or abattoir workers may be exposed to this organism that is responsible for a chronic flu-like illness. Conjunctivitis is an important clue to the diagnosis as are the multiple segmental opacities on the chest X-ray.

5. **B. *Chlamydia psittaci*.** Psittacosis presents as a chronic illness in those exposed to birds carrying the organism (e.g. pet-shop workers). The hepatosplenomegaly and patchy lower lobe consolidation make this a more likely cause of the low-grade pyrexia than the other organisms in the option list.

TUBERCULOSIS

4.12 **For each of the following patients with tuberculosis (TB), select the most appropriate clinical description.**

A   Aspergilloma
B   Cryptic miliary TB
C   Miliary TB
D   Phlyctenular conjunctivitis
E   Post-primary pulmonary TB
F   Renal TB
G   Tuberculous Addison's disease
H   Tuberculous enteritis
I   Tuberculous meningitis
J   Tuberculous pyopneumothorax

1. A 17-year-old man presents with a 2-week history of general malaise, night sweats, weight loss and mild shortness of breath. He has a high temperature, hepatosplenomegaly and evidence of choroidal tubercles on ophthalmoscopy. Investigations reveal that he is anaemic but the chest X-ray, mid-stream urine (MSU) and sputum cultures are all normal.

2. A 42-year-old woman presents with a 3-month history of cough productive of yellow sputum. She has lost 8 kg in weight and feels generally unwell. On examination, there are persistent crackles in the right upper zone. The chest X-ray shows an ill-defined opacity in the right upper lobe and a small pleural effusion.

3. A 50-year-old man presents with night sweats, weight loss and anaemia. The chest X-ray shows a small calcified nodule in the right upper lobe. Sputum culture is normal and the MSU shows no red cells, 500 white cells and no organisms on Gram stain.

4. A 20-year-old woman is admitted as an emergency complaining of headache, photophobia and neck stiffness. The chest X-ray is normal. A lumbar puncture is performed and microscopy of the CSF shows a lymphocytosis; the CSF glucose is 0.5 mmol/L and the plasma glucose is 7.8 mmol/L. Ziehl–Neelsen staining of the CSF is negative.

5. An 81-year-old woman is admitted with a history of general deterioration. She is frail with a low-grade pyrexia. Chest X-ray, sputum, urine and blood cultures are all normal. She has an appropriate response to synacthen. She continues to deteriorate and dies. At post mortem, acid and alcohol-fast bacilli are cultured from the liver, lungs, bone marrow and spleen.

Answers to 4.12

1. **C. Miliary TB.** The history may be relatively short and there are often few signs or symptoms in the chest. It may be difficult to isolate bacilli from cultures. Choroidal tubercles and hepatosplenomegaly help to make the diagnosis in this case.

2. **E. Post-primary pulmonary TB.** The relatively long history and chest X-ray findings in this woman makes re-activation of previous TB the most likely cause of her illness.

3. **F. Renal TB.** Sterile pyuria should always raise the suspicion of renal TB.

4. **I. Tuberculous meningitis.** This is a rare condition in the UK but still an important cause of death in young adults elsewhere in the world. The important finding is a very low CSF sugar in the presence of a lymphocytosis.

5. **B. Cryptic miliary TB.** The patient has miliary TB since bacilli have been cultured from a number of sites. She does not have Addison's disease, since the synacthen test is normal. It is 'cryptic' because there were few, if any, clues to the diagnosis before death.

INTERSTITIAL LUNG DISEASE

4.13 **For each of the following patients with interstitial lung disease, select the most likely diagnosis.**

A   Alveolar microlithiasis
B   Alveolar proteinosis
C   Byssinosis
D   Cheese worker's lung
E   Histiocytosis X
F   Idiopathic pulmonary haemosiderosis
G   Lymphangioleiomyomatosis
H   Neurofibromatosis
I   Non-cardiogenic pulmonary oedema
J   Pulmonary eosinophilia

1.   A 70-year-old man complains of shortness of breath on exertion and a dry cough. The chest X-ray shows diffuse calcified micronodular shadowing, more pronounced in the lower lobes.

2.   A 36-year-old woman complains of shortness of breath on exertion and haemoptysis. Clinically she has a pleural effusion and when it is tapped, milky fluid is obtained. The chest X-ray and thoracic CT scan show thin-walled cysts throughout both lungs and a moderate-sized effusion.

3.   A 42-year-old man has been seeing his general practitioner for the last 2 years with poorly controlled hypertension. He complains of shortness of breath, a dry cough and episodes of palpitations. His chest X-ray shows bilateral reticular nodular shadowing.

4.   A 7-year-old boy is taken to A&E after coughing up blood. He has been short of breath for several months and looks pale. The chest X-ray shows bilateral perihilar infiltrates and a CT scan reveals diffuse pulmonary fibrosis.

5.   A 22-year-old man is found collapsed outside a night-club and taken to hospital. On examination, he is unrousable, has pin-point pupils and a respiratory rate of 4 breaths/min. The chest X-ray shows widespread intra-alveolar shadowing.

Answers to 4.13

1. **A. Alveolar microlithiasis.** This is a rare disorder but the micronodular calcification is characteristic. Treatment with disodium etidronate has been suggested. Previous measles pneumonia can also lead to multiple calcified nodules on the chest X-ray.

2. **G. Lymphangioleiomyomatosis.** This is the only option in the list that may cause a chylous effusion. This is a rare disease of women, usually of childbearing age. There is proliferation of benign, atypical smooth muscle cells in the walls of the lymphatics of the lower respiratory tract. The clinical findings include dyspnoea, recurrent chylous pleural effusions, pneumothorax and haemoptysis.

3. **H. Neurofibromatosis.** The poorly controlled hypertension and palpitations are the clue to the diagnosis. Neurofibromas may occur in the skin and most other organs. Diffuse interstitial fibrosis in the lungs causes the reticular nodular shadowing on the chest X-ray.

4. **F. Idiopathic pulmonary haemosiderosis.** This is a slowly progressive disorder in adults, but in children it can progress very rapidly. The patients present with dyspnoea, haemoptysis and anaemia. Death may occur from massive pulmonary haemorrhage.

5. **I. Non-cardiogenic pulmonary oedema.** The patient has signs of narcosis, i.e. small pupils and a depressed respiratory rate. The chest X-ray is in keeping with pulmonary oedema, a well-recognized adverse effect of opiates. The patient had taken intravenous diamorphine in the club and had collapsed on leaving.

MANAGEMENT OF CHEST DISEASES

4.14 **For each of the following patients who present with respiratory symptoms, select the most appropriate treatment.**

A Continuous positive airways pressure (CPAP) ventilation
B High volume oxygen
C Intravenous antibiotics
D Long-term domiciliary oxygen
E Nebulized steroids
F Occasional bronchodilator as required
G Oral antibiotics
H Regular inhaled steroids
I Single lung transplantation
J Systemic steroids

1. A 17-year-old student visits his general practitioner complaining of shortness of breath and wheezing lasting several hours after attending a bonfire party. On direct questioning, he recalls feeling wheezy occasionally in very dusty environments.

2. A 19-year-old woman visits her general practitioner complaining of shortness of breath and wheeze after exercise. She is often troubled by a non-productive cough at night.

3. A 72-year-old woman is seen in the Chest Clinic with a 5-year history of increasing shortness of breath on exertion. She has smoked for many years. On examination, she is thin and tachypnoeic but not cyanosed. Her chest appears hyperexpanded but auscultation is unremarkable. While breathing air, her arterial blood gases show a Po_2 of 6 kPa (normal 12–15), but a normal Pco_2, pH and [HCO_3^-]. After 1h of breathing 28% oxygen via a mask, her Po_2 rises to 8 kPa and the Pco_2 remains normal.

4. A 60-year-old factory worker visits his general practitioner complaining of a 3-day history of shortness of breath and cough productive of green sputum. He is a non-smoker and has been previously fit and well. On examination, he is pyrexial and tachypnoeic. Percussion of the chest is normal but there are some expiratory crackles at the left base.

5. A 35-year-old teacher is admitted complaining of a 2-day history of shortness of breath. On the morning of admission, she developed sharp left-sided chest pain and started coughing up rusty-coloured sputum. She is pyrexial, mildly cyanosed, has herpes labialis and is tachypnoeic. There is reduced expansion of the right lower chest wall, with dullness to percussion, crackles and bronchial breathing at the right base.

Answers to 4.14

1. **F. Occasional bronchodilator as required.** This young man gives a history of airway irritability and is likely to have asthma. However, he has symptoms only when exposed to uncommon situations so he does not need continuous, regular treatment.

2. **H. Regular inhaled steroids.** This woman has asthma with regular symptoms including nocturnal symptoms. Apart from a regular inhaled bronchodilator, she should take an inhaled steroid every day (typically morning and night). This will reduce the frequency of acute attacks.

3. **D. Long-term domiciliary oxygen.** The patient has chronic type 1 respiratory failure and clinically is a 'pink puffer'. She does not retain CO_2 following a trial of oxygen and the low Po_2 fulfils the current guidelines for the use of long-term domiciliary oxygen. She should stop smoking for her own health and also to reduce the risk of fire. Survival benefit has been shown if the oxygen is used for at least 15 h/day.

4. **G. Oral antibiotics.** The use of antibiotics for chest symptoms in general practice is a controversial area. In the main, they are still over-prescribed and are over-demanded by patients, most of whom will get better without them. Nevertheless, patients with chest signs on examination may benefit although it should be noted that pyrexia, shortness of breath and even green sputum are more commonly viral in origin. In this case, oral antibiotics are certainly more appropriate than any of the other options.

5. **C. Intravenous antibiotics.** The history and examination are typical of an acute lobar pneumonia. Her systemic symptoms, tachypnoea and cyanosis suggest a moderately severe pneumonia and most authorities would use intravenous antibiotics for at least the first 24 h of therapy. Herpes labialis is often seen in patients with pneumococcal pneumonia.

5

Gastrointestinal and hepatobiliary systems

GASTROINTESTINAL POLYPS

5.1 For each of the following patients with gastrointestinal polyps, select the most likely diagnosis.

A   Colorectal cancer
B   Cowden's disease
C   Crohn's disease
D   Cronkhite–Canada syndrome
E   Familial adenomatous polyposis
F   Juvenile polyposis
G   Peutz–Jeghers syndrome
H   Sporadic tubular adenoma
I   Sporadic villous adenoma
J   Ulcerative colitis

1. A patient with many gastric and colonic polyps who also has alopecia, cutaneous hyperpigmentation and nail dystrophy. There is no family history.

2. A patient with multiple polyps in the small intestine who also has multiple dark spots around the lips. Her mother also has the condition.

3. A patient with a history of abdominal pain, rectal bleeding and anaemia has hundreds of mucus-filled polyps in the rectum, colon and duodenum. His father died of carcinoma of the colon when he was 26 years of age.

4. A patient with hundreds of polyps in the rectum, colon and stomach also has dark round pigmented retinal lesions.

5. A patient with hypokalaemia and a single sessile lesion in the sigmoid colon.

Answers to 5.1

1.　**D. Cronkhite–Canada syndrome.** There is no family history, which makes this a more likely diagnosis than the other polyposis syndromes listed. In addition, the patient has hair loss, pigmentation and nail dystrophy which are also associated with this diagnosis.

2.　**G. Peutz–Jeghers syndrome.** The family history and the melanin pigmentation around the lips together with the small intestinal polyps should point to this as the correct diagnosis.

3.　**F. Juvenile polyposis.** The patient's symptoms and family history of cancer at a young age is suggestive of juvenile polyposis. The clue to the correct diagnosis here is the fact that the polyps (which are hamartomas) are filled with mucus. Up to 20% of sufferers develop carcinoma of the colon before the age of 40 years.

4.　**E. Familial adenomatous polyposis.** Congenital hypertrophy of the retinal pigment epithelium is seen in about two-thirds of patients and is an important phenotypic marker for the disease. It is an autosomal dominant condition and all at-risk relatives with retinal lesions will also have gastrointestinal polyposis. Symptoms may be minimal but malignant transformation is inevitable.

5.　**I. Sporadic villous adenoma.** This is among the causes of hypokalaemia because of the secretion of profuse amounts of mucus leading to loss of potassium.

INVESTIGATION OF GASTROINTESTINAL DISEASE

5.2 **For each of the following clinical scenarios, select the most appropriate investigation.**

A Barium enema
B Barium follow-through
C Barium meal
D Barium swallow
E Colonoscopy
F Enteroscopy
G Gastrografin enema
H Oesophago-gastro-duodenoscopy
I Plain abdominal film
J Rigid sigmoidoscopy

1. A 68-year-old man presents with a 3-month history of dysphagia and has lost 10 kg in weight.

2. A 36-year-old woman presents with acute iritis. Her medical history includes recurrent episodes of abdominal pain and initial investigations show her to have an iron deficient anaemia.

3. A 38-year-old man presents with loose motions, containing blood but no mucus. He has a 12-year history of ulcerative colitis but has not been a regular attendee to the out-patient clinic. On examination, he is thin but otherwise looks reasonably well. The abdomen is not distended but there is mild tenderness in the left iliac fossa.

4. A 76-year-old woman is admitted to hospital in a confused state. On examination, she is dehydrated, the abdomen is distended and there is generalized tenderness, guarding and rebound tenderness.

5. A 45-year-old man is admitted after a small haematemesis. Apart from the patient looking thin, examination is unremarkable. He volunteers that he has lost 5 kg in weight over the last 6 weeks. Initial investigations reveal that he has an iron deficiency anaemia.

Answers to 5.2

1. **D. Barium swallow.** This is the investigation of choice for a patient with dysphagia, since one would need to know whether there is any compression of the oesophagus and, if there is, whether it is intrinsic or extrinsic (e.g. lymph nodes, retrosternal goitre). Loss of weight is a sinister sign and carcinoma of the oesophagus is a likely diagnosis.

2. **B. Barium follow-through.** The history is suggestive of Crohn's disease (iritis, recurrent abdominal pain and anaemia). A follow-through examination will allow visualization of the proximal small intestine that may show features of patchy involvement.

3. **E. Colonoscopy.** The patient has had ulcerative colitis for more than 10 years and is at high risk of colonic malignancy. The colon should be adequately visualized with a technique that will also allow biopsies to be taken.

4. **I. Plain abdominal film.** In practice, a plain abdominal film is often the first investigation in a patient with an acute abdomen. The history in this woman suggests that she may have a perforated intra-abdominal viscus. An erect chest X-ray is also requested as this may show free-air under the diaphragm more clearly than on the abdominal films.

5. **H. Oesophago-gastro-duodenoscopy.** The history is suggestive of a possible gastric malignancy and an upper-GI endoscopy should be performed in the near future.

GASTROINTESTINAL TRACT INFECTIONS

5.3 **For each of the following patients with infection in the gastrointestinal tract, select the most likely causative organism.**

A   *Campylobacter jejuni*
B   *Clostridium difficile*
C   *E. coli O157*
D   *Entamoeba histolytica*
E   *Giardia lamblia*
F   *Helicobacter pylori*
G   Rotavirus
H   *Strongyloides stercoralis*
I   *Tuberculosis bovis*
J   *Yersinia*

1.   A 22-year-old student returns from a visit to St Petersburg. Two weeks later, he complains of abdominal pain, diarrhoea, anorexia and nausea. On examination, his abdomen is distended and tender. Stools are reported as showing a scanty number of cysts.

2.   A 30-year-old man returns from the tropics. Six months later, he attends his general practitioner complaining of altered bowel habit, occasional episodes of diarrhoea with blood-streaking of the stools alternating with periods of constipation. On examination, he is tender in the right iliac fossa. Initial stool cultures are negative but fresh samples show trophozoites under the light microscope.

3.   A 32-year-old woman suddenly develops diarrhoea and vomiting. She had been feeling perfectly well before the attack. The symptoms last 36 h and then completely resolve.

4.   A 40-year-old woman returns after a period of time working in the Far East. She is referred to a hospital out-patient clinic because over the next month she develops abdominal bloating and pain associated with bulky, offensive stools that are difficult to flush away. Under the light microscope, stool samples contain no cysts or ova but mobile larvae.

5.   A 22-year-old man is admitted to hospital following a haematemesis. Oesophago-gastro-duodenoscopy shows a duodenal ulcer. In the past, he has had episodes of epigastric pain and indigestion which responded to antacids.

Answers to 5.3

1. **E.** *Giardia lamblia.* Cysts remain viable in water for several months and this is the main source of spread. It is common in the tropics but St Petersburg (formerly Leningrad) developed notoriety as a city in which to catch the infection after several outbreaks in recent years.

2. **D.** *Entamoeba histolytica.* This is common in the tropics and an important cause to consider in travellers returning from the area. Typically, it runs a chronic course. The trophozoites are best seen when mobile and this will only be in fresh, warm stool.

3. **G. Rotavirus.** Rapid onset of self-limiting diarrhoea and vomiting is either viral in origin or due to the ingestion of toxin-producing bacteria. Rotaviruses cause epidemics of diarrhoea and vomiting in nurseries and schools.

4. **H.** *Strongyloides stercoralis.* This is a small nematode that is common in the Far East. It parasitizes and damages the jejunal mucosa leading to malabsorption. The larvae are intermittently passed in the stools but repeated examinations may be required before the diagnosis is made.

5. **F.** *Helicobacter pylori.* Over 90% of duodenal ulcers in young patients are associated with *H. pylori* and successful eradication of the infection results in a much reduced relapse rate when compared to the administration of proton pump inhibitors alone.

MALABSORPTION

5.4 **For each of the following patients with malabsorption, select the most likely diagnosis.**

A   Bacterial overgrowth
B   Chronic alcoholic pancreatitis
C   Coeliac disease
D   Crohn's disease
E   Cystic fibrosis
F   Giardiasis
G   HIV enteropathy
H   Lactase deficiency
I   Tropical sprue
J   Whipple's disease

1.   A 46-year-old man is being investigated for generalized lymphadenopathy. He complains of aching in his joints and lethargy. A full blood count reveals he is anaemic so he undergoes an upper gastrointestinal endoscopy. Duodenal biopsies are reported as showing numerous macrophages in the lamina propria.

2.   A 24-year-old woman is seen by her general practitioner because she is having difficulty conceiving. She is noted to be thin and pale and admits to a several-year history of intermittent diarrhoea and weight loss. A full blood count reveals she is anaemic with a macrocytosis. An upper gastrointestinal endoscopy is normal but a barium follow-through study shows multiple small-bowel strictures.

3.   A 40-year-old man has been admitted to hospital on several occasions with chest infections. He has never smoked, although he recalls having a 'weak chest' as a child. During his last admission, he was found to have diabetes and was started on insulin. He has become increasingly underweight over the last 2 years and cannot put on any more weight. On direct questioning, he admits to having diarrhoea, passing large and bulky stools.

4.   A 27-year-old woman seeks advice because she has developed diarrhoea over the last 3 months. On examination, she has an itchy, blistering rash over her elbows. Biochemical investigations show that she has low serum albumin, calcium and folate concentrations.

5.   A 56-year-old man with a long history of chronic epigastric and back pain is referred to the local hospital with newly-diagnosed diabetes. On direct questioning, he reports a 9-month history of weight loss and steatorrhoea. His full blood count is normal apart from a macrocytosis.

Answers to 5.4

1. **J. Whipple's disease.** Although the generalized lymphadenopathy may have initially suggested HIV enteropathy, the arthropathy is typical of Whipple's disease. The macrophages contain glycoprotein that stains with the periodic acid Schiff (PAS) reagent.

2. **D. Crohn's disease.** The important investigation in this case is the barium follow-through that shows the small-bowel strictures typical of Crohn's. The macrocytosis is due to vitamin B_{12} malabsorption as a result of the Crohn's disease affecting the terminal ileum where the B_{12}-intrinsic factor complex is normally absorbed.

3. **E. Cystic fibrosis.** With the discovery of the cystic fibrosis gene, it is now recognized that some people have mutations that present with relatively mild features in childhood but cause problems in later life. This is sometimes called 'late-onset cystic fibrosis'. The recurrent chest infections in this patient raised suspicions, especially as he was a non-smoker and there was no family history of asthma. Both endocrine (leading to diabetes) and exocrine (leading to malabsorption) pancreatic failure are features of cystic fibrosis.

4. **C. Coeliac disease.** This disorder may present at any age, even in the elderly. It is due to hypersensitivity to the gliadin component of cereals. The rash in this case is dermatitis herpetiformis, a marker of the disease.

5. **B. Chronic alcoholic pancreatitis.** Although no alcohol history is given, the epigastric and back pain is suggestive of chronic pancreatitis. Bacterial overgrowth may occur in diabetes, but it is relatively uncommon and tends to be a late complication in patients with autonomic neuropathy and the consequential disordered small intestinal motility. The macrocytosis is a further pointer to the excessive alcohol ingestion of this patient.

DISORDERS OF THE LOWER GASTROINTESTINAL TRACT

5.5 **For each of the following patients with disorders of the lower gastrointestinal tract, select the most likely diagnosis.**

A   Acquired megacolon
B   Anal fissure
C   Colonic pseudo-obstruction
D   Diverticulitis
E   Diverticulosis
F   Haemorrhoids
G   Hirschsprung's disease
H   Melanosis coli
I   Pruritus ani
J   Solitary rectal ulcer

1.   A 22-year-old man complains of irregular bowel motions with occasional bleeding and mucus per rectum. Sigmoidoscopy reveals a lesion on the anterior rectal wall and biopsies show an accumulation of collagen but no evidence of malignancy.

2.   A 60-year-old woman complains of altered bowel habit. Sigmoidoscopy is normal but a barium enema reveals out-pouchings of the mucosa in the sigmoid colon.

3.   A 54-year-old woman complains of severe chronic constipation despite the regular use of many laxatives. Sigmoidoscopy reveals a 'tiger-skin' discoloration of the colonic mucosa.

4.   A 62-year-old man complains of severe left iliac fossa pain. On examination, he is pyrexial and there is abdominal tenderness with guarding and rebound tenderness.

5.   A 17-year-old woman with a history of constipation complains of severe pain on opening her bowels. There is a little blood on the toilet paper when she wipes herself. She refuses to be examined.

Answers to 5.5

1. **J. Solitary rectal ulcer.** This is most common in young adults and the cause is largely unknown although chronic trauma due to constipation may play a role. Sigmoidoscopy will show an ulcer which may look like a carcinoma but histology is diagnostic showing inflammatory changes, bands of smooth muscle extending into the lamina propria and the accumulation of collagen. Blood or mucus per rectum and tenesmus are associated symptoms.

2. **E. Diverticulosis.** This is a common finding on barium enema and is asymptomatic. Another cause for the altered bowel habit should be sought.

3. **H. Melanosis coli.** Long-term abuse of stimulant laxatives may lead to an accumulation of melanin pigment in macrophages of the lamina propria. The normal pink appearance is altered by streaks of pigmentation. The inside of the rectum may have a speckled appearance with many pinkish spots that have escaped pigmentation. This appearance is characteristic in patients who have taken large quantities of anthracene laxatives and it may betray factitious diarrhoea. This should not be confused with the 'brown bowel syndrome' (found in steatorrhoea) in which there is lipofuscin deposition in myocytes.

4. **D. Diverticulitis.** *Note* that acute inflammation in diverticulosis is diverticulitis.

5. **B. Anal fissure.** Severe pain on opening the bowels suggests a local cause.

INVESTIGATION OF HEPATOBILIARY DISEASE

5.6 **For each of the following patients in whom a hepatobiliary disease is suspected, select the least invasive investigation most likely to help in the diagnosis.**

A Australia antigen
B Endoscopic retrograde cholangiopancreatography (ERCP)
C Liver biopsy
D Serum α-fetoprotein
E Serum anti-mitochondrial antibodies
F Serum anti-smooth muscle antibodies
G Serum caeruloplasmin
H Serum ferritin
I Splenic biopsy
J Ultrasound of portal vein

1. A 52-year-old man with diabetes and hypogonadism is referred to a hospital clinic because he has abnormal liver function tests.

2. A 17-year-old woman under the care of a psychiatrist is noted to have apparently involuntary movements. Biochemical tests show her to have abnormal liver function tests.

3. A 48-year-old man with known alcoholic liver disease is admitted to hospital after developing abdominal pain and tense ascites.

4. A 43-year-old woman with a 12-month history of pruritus is found to have cholestatic liver function test results.

5. A 52-year-old man who has been drinking at least 60 units of alcohol a week for the last 10 years is admitted to hospital with recurrent attacks of abdominal pain, intermittent jaundice and raised serum amylase.

Answers to 5.6

1.   **H. Serum ferritin.** The patient may have haemochromatosis.

2.   **G. Serum caeruloplasmin.** The patient may have Wilson's disease.

3.   **D. Serum α-fetoprotein.** Decompensation of chronic liver disease may occur with the development of a hepatocellular carcinoma.

4.   **E. Serum anti-mitochondrial antibodies.** The patient may have primary biliary cirrhosis.

5.   **B. ERCP.** The patient may have chronic pancreatitis.

HEPATITIS

5.7 **For each of the following patients with hepatitis, select the most likely diagnosis.**

Normal values: bilirubin <17 mmol/L, ALT 5–35 IU, alkaline phosphatase 30–300 IU.

A   Autoimmune hepatitis
B   Cytomegalovirus infection
C   Hepatitis A
D   Hepatitis B
E   Hepatitis C
F   Hepatitis D
G   Hepatitis E
H   Infectious mononucleosis
I   Kalar-azar
J   Primary biliary cirrhosis

1. A 58-year-old woman is seen by her general practitioner complaining of generalized pruritus. The liver function tests show an alkaline phosphatase of 1074 IU, bilirubin of 24 mmol/L, ALT of 26 IU. Anti-mitochondrial antibodies are present at a titre of 1:640.

2. A 14-year-old boy with Down's syndrome living in an institution is seen by his general practitioner with a flu-like illness. Four days later, the doctor is called again because the boy has become jaundiced.

3. A 21-year-old male student is seen by his general practitioner with right upper quadrant tenderness, nausea and sore throat. He is given a course of amoxicillin but the following day develops a florid macular rash over his arms, legs, chest and back. On examination, he has moderate splenomegaly and is mildly jaundiced.

4. A 50-year-old man with known chronic hepatitis B infection presents with jaundice, mild ascites and hepatic encephalopathy. His liver function tests show an AST of 2100 IU, and a bilirubin of 96 mmol/L.

5. A 21-year-old woman who is known to inject illicit drugs intravenously presents with a flu-like illness. Her liver function tests show an AST of 126, Hepatitis B virus surface antigen negative and hepatitis B virus surface antibody positive.

Answers to 5.7

1. **J. Primary biliary cirrhosis.** This disorder is most common in middle-aged women and associated with the presence of anti-mitochondrial antibodies. Pruritus is a common presentation.

2. **C. Hepatitis A.** This commonly presents as a flu-like illness followed by jaundice and is spread by the faecal-oral route. Many cases are asymptomatic.

3. **H. Infectious mononucleosis.** Infection with the Epstein–Barr virus results in this condition, also termed glandular fever. Hepatosplenomegaly and jaundice occur only in a minority of affected individuals. The reaction to amoxicillin is typical. A transient rash is typical and occurs in about 90% of patients who receive this drug for a viral sore throat. This is one reason why antibiotics should not be prescribed to people with suspected viral infections.

4. **F. Hepatitis D.** Infection with hepatitis D may supervene in patients who already have chronic hepatitis B infection.

5. **E. Hepatitis C.** This woman has been vaccinated against hepatitis B, hence the presence of antibody against the hepatitis B surface antibody and the absence of antigen. Hepatitis C is an increasingly prevalent infection in the intravenous drug-abusing community.

LESIONS IN THE HEPATOBILIARY SYSTEM

5.8 **For each of the following patients with hepatobiliary disease, select the most likely cause.**

A   Adult hepatorenal polycystic disease
B   Choledochal cysts
C   Congenital hepatic fibrosis
D   Focal nodular hyperplasia of the liver
E   Hepatic adenoma
F   Hepatocellular carcinoma
G   Hydatid cyst of the liver
H   Nodular regenerative hyperplasia of the liver
I   Pyogenic liver abscess
J   Veno-occlusive disease of the liver

1. A 76-year-old retired Welsh farmer with hereditary haemochromatosis is found to have a 3×4 cm mass in the right lobe of the liver on ultrasound and a raised serum α-fetoprotein.

2. A 31-year-old English housewife with right upper quadrant pain is found to have an 8×4 cm mass in the left lobe of the liver on ultrasound. She is on no medication apart from paracetamol for the pain and the oral contraceptive pill.

3. A 56-year-old Irish farmer with right upper quadrant pain is found to have a large, smooth and non-tender mass in the right upper quadrant on examination. Plain abdominal X-rays show a heavily calcified mass.

4. A 10-year-old Japanese girl has had several episodes of right upper quadrant pain. On examination, she is mildly icteric. An ERCP shows multiple cystic lesions communicating with the common bile duct.

5. A 68-year-old professional gardener presents with weight loss, night sweats, jaundice and swinging pyrexia. Her medical history includes type 2 diabetes and diverticular disease. Abdominal ultrasound shows multiple masses in the liver.

Answers to 5.8

1. **F. Hepatocellular carcinoma.** This may develop in cirrhotic liver, such as that found in haemochromatosis. α-fetoprotein is a tumour marker for this malignancy.

2. **E. Hepatic adenoma.** These are incidental findings that usually cause no symptoms but are associated with use of the oral contraceptive pill.

3. **G. Hydatid cyst of the liver.** Livestock farmers who may be exposed to hydatid can present with advanced disease. Typically, the hydatid cyst shows heavy calcification.

4. **B. Choledochal cysts.** This is an uncommon condition but the description given is characteristic. It has been reported more frequently in the Japanese and other Asian races and in 80% of cases, the patient is female. Many patients will be asymptomatic but some may develop biliary peritonitis from a ruptured cyst.

5. **I. Pyogenic liver abscess.** The history is suggestive of an infective disease process, with pyrexia, night sweats and weight loss. About one-third of patients are jaundiced on presentation. The multiple pyogenic abscesses may have arisen from an episode of diverticulitis. Ultrasonography is helpful but in many cases the abscesses are small and are not detected.

Urogenital system

DRUGS AND THE KIDNEY

6.1 **For each of the following disorders affecting the urinary tract, select the most likely causative agent.**

A   Acyclovir
B   Angiotensin-converting enzyme inhibitor
C   Gold injections
D   L-DOPA
E   Lead
F   Methysergide
G   Non-steroidal anti-inflammatory drug (NSAID)
H   Paracetamol
I   Quinine bisulphate
J   Rosiglitazone

1.   Interstitial nephritis.

2.   Acute tubular necrosis.

3.   Retroperitoneal fibrosis.

4.   Obstructive uropathy due to crystal deposition.

5.   Membranous nephropathy.

Answers to 6.1

1. **G. Non-steroidal anti-inflammatory drug (NSAID).** Interstitial nephritis has been reported with most NSAIDs.

2. **H. Paracetamol.** Although acute tubular necrosis can supervene following adverse reactions to many drugs, clinically the most common problem is in patients who develop hepato-renal failure following overdosage of paracetamol.

3. **F. Methysergide.** This drug is still occasionally used in the treatment of resistant migraine.

4. **A. Acyclovir.** Renal function should be carefully monitored in all patients receiving acyclovir and dehydration should be avoided to reduce the risk of crystal deposition.

5. **C. Gold injections.** Gold therapy is used in the treatment of rheumatoid arthritis. Patients with rheumatoid disease may develop renal failure for a variety of causes including the use of drugs such as NSAIDs. Urinalysis for proteinuria should be part of the regular follow-up of patients taking gold.

INVESTIGATIONS IN RENAL DISEASE

6.2 **For each of the following patients with renal disease, select the investigation that is most likely to yield a diagnosis.**

A   CT scan
B   DMSA scan
C   DTPA scan
D   Intravenous urogram
E   Micturating cystourethrography
F   MRI scan
G   Plain abdominal X-ray
H   Renal arteriogram
I   Renal biopsy
J   Renal ultrasound

1. A 40-year-old woman is referred to the medical out-patient department because she has developed persistent hypertension that is responding poorly to treatment. On direct questioning, she recalls having been treated for several urinary tract infections as a teenager. Her MSU and plasma urea and electrolytes are normal.

2. A 21-year-old man has had type 1 diabetes for the last 2 years. He is seen sooner than planned in the diabetes clinic because he has developed swelling of the legs and face. Urine dip-stick shows glucose +, ketones +, protein +++, blood +.

3. A 60-year-old man consults his general practitioner after passing blood in his urine. Initial biochemical investigations show that he has hypercalcaemia. While he is waiting to be seen in a hospital clinic, he develops severe loin pain, dysuria and haematuria and he is admitted urgently to hospital.

4. A 56-year-old man is admitted to hospital as an emergency complaining of severe colicky abdominal pain. Urine dip-stick testing shows blood +++, protein –, glucose –.

5. A 72-year-old man with long-standing type 2 diabetes and poorly controlled hypertension is commenced on captopril. He returns 10 days later complaining of nausea and vomiting. His plasma urea has risen from 8.0 to 54 and his creatinine from 142 to 870.

Answers to 6.2

1.   **J. Renal ultrasound.** The hypertension may be secondary to renal scarring produced by the recurrent urinary tract infections. A renal ultrasound may also reveal predisposing factors for infections such as duplex ureters.

2.   **I. Renal biopsy.** The diabetes has not been present long enough to make diabetic nephropathy a likely cause of this man's nephrotic syndrome. Although a renal ultrasound must be performed prior to the renal biopsy, it is the biopsy that is most likely to yield the final diagnosis.

3.   **D. Intravenous urogram.** The history is one of renal stones. A renal ultrasound may show a dilated renal tract or stones and a stone may be seen on a plain abdominal film. However, an intravenous urogram was required in this patient to detect a small stone that had lodged at the point where the right ureter enters the pelvic brim.

4.   **G. Plain abdominal X-ray.** This man is likely to be passing a renal stone. The first imaging investigation should be a plain X-ray since many renal stones are radio-opaque and may be seen lying along the line of the ureter. An ultrasound or IVU may be required subsequently.

5.   **H. Renal arteriogram.** The patient had renal artery stenosis and this explains the deterioration in renal function after the use of the angiotensin-converting enzyme inhibitor, captopril. Spiral CT and MRI scanning may supersede the traditional renal arteriogram in the future and would be acceptable answers in situations where there is the suitable expertise.

ABNORMALITIES OF THE URINE

6.3   For each of the following patients with altered urine colour, select the most likely diagnosis.

A   Alkaptonuria
B   Anthocyanins
C   Anthraquinones
D   Haemoglobinuria
E   L-DOPA
F   Macroscopic haematuria
G   Microscopic haematuria
H   Myoglobinuria
I   Porphyria
J   Rifampicin

1.   A 62-year-old man with severe right-sided loin pain that radiates to the groin.

2.   A 28-year-old woman who complains of passing orange-coloured urine after consuming large quantities of senna.

3.   A 34-year-old woman is admitted to a surgical ward complaining of severe abdominal pain. The nursing staff notice that the urine becomes dark red while the sample is left in the sluice, awaiting collection.

4.   A 40-year-old woman complains of passing red urine after commencing treatment for tuberculosis.

5.   A 28-year-old man is admitted to the trauma ward after being rescued from under a collapsed wall. His urine is noticed to be almost black in colour.

Answers to 6.3

1. **F. Macroscopic haematuria.** The man is passing a renal stone.

2. **C. Anthraquinones.** Senna contains anthraquinones that turn urine an orange colour. Beetroot turns the urine red and contains anthocyanins.

3. **I. Porphyria.** This woman has acute intermittent porphyria. Levels of the porphyrin precursors, delta-amino laevulinic acid (ALA) and porphobilinogen (PBG), are markedly raised in the urine during an acute attack. PBG turns reddish-brown on standing and can be detected with the use of Ehrlich's aldehyde reagent. Levels may also be moderately elevated between attacks.

4. **J. Rifampicin.** Patients given rifampicin in the treatment of tuberculosis or as prophylaxis against meningococcal meningitis should be warned that their body fluids will become transiently discoloured.

5. **H. Myoglobinuria.** Rhabdomyolysis following a crush injury causes very dark, mahogany-coloured urine. Renal failure may supervene.

DISORDERS OF THE KIDNEY AND URINARY TRACT

6.4 **Select the most likely diagnosis requiring further investigation in each of the following clinical presentations.**

A Acute pyelonephritis
B Benign hypertrophy of the prostate
C Diabetic nephropathy
D Nephroblastoma
E Nephrocalcinosis
F Polyarteritis nodosa
G Pyonephrosis
H Renal carcinoma
I Renal tuberculosis
J Retroperitoneal fibrosis

1. A 42-year-old obese housewife presents with a recurrent dull pain in her loins for the last 4 months. Fourteen months ago, she had an ileo-jejunal bypass operation for her obesity and hypercholesterolaemia. Before the operation, she weighed 160 kg and she is now 102 kg. Her urine contains protein and red blood cells.

2. A 38-year-old housewife developed a pain in her right loin that radiated to the corresponding iliac fossa and the suprapubic region. During the next day, she vomited four times. She has dysuria, fever, rigors and there is tenderness in both loins.

3. A 68-year-old retired teacher has developed increased frequency of micturition for the last 3 months. He has precipitancy and cannot hold his water for long, and when he does pass it, he dribbles and cannot make a stream. He has had two episodes of urinary tract infection.

4. A 55-year-old policeman has had low back pain for the last 6 months. He spent a few weeks off work because of malaise, anorexia and fever. He has lost 10 kg in weight. His general practitioner found that his serum urea was elevated at 20 mmol/L. A renal ultrasound shows bilaterally enlarged kidneys.

5. A 22-year-old unemployed man has had vague symptoms of malaise and lethargy for the last 9 months. He has had frequent night sweats and has lost 6 kg in weight. His urine, tested twice a fortnight apart, contained red and white blood cells but grew no organisms.

Answers to 6.4

1. **E. Nephrocalcinosis.** A well-recognized complication of this procedure is nephrocalcinosis due to oxalate deposition. Oxalate is produced by the overpopulation of bacteria in the blind loop and is absorbed excessively by the short segment of the functional jejunum. The urine and blood should be tested for the oxalate concentration.

2. **A. Acute pyelonephritis.** The dysuria, fever and rigors suggest urinary tract infection. The urine should be tested for the presence of pus cells and organisms and an intravenous pyelogram should be arranged to look for any stones and assess the function of the kidneys.

3. **B. Benign hypertrophy of the prostate.** The symptomatology suggests urinary outflow tract obstruction, most probably caused by an enlarged prostate. A per rectum examination would be an essential part of the clinical examination in this setting. An intravenous pyelogram would be necessary before any operative procedure is contemplated.

4. **J. Retroperitoneal fibrosis.** This diagnosis should be borne in mind when a middle-aged man with unexplained uraemia presents with low back pain, low-grade fever and loss of weight. Pain is the most common symptom but it is rather vague. An intravenous pyelogram is an important initial investigation as it might show displacement of the ureters towards the midline and obstruction at the pelvic brim. Magnetic resonance imaging will help to identify the retroperitoneal fibrotic mass but it cannot help to distinguish it from a tumour. A laparotomy will be the ultimate investigative and therapeutic procedure and multiple biopsies should be taken to explore the nature of the mass.

5. **I. Renal tuberculosis.** A clinical setting of night sweats, recurrent haematuria and sterile pyuria must alert the clinician about the possibility of renal tuberculosis. Urine should be cultured for tubercle bacilli and a cystoscopic examination should be carried out to visualize the urinary bladder for the presence of any granulomata.

GLOMERULONEPHRITIS

6.5 **For each of the following patients with glomerulonephritis, select the most likely diagnosis.**

A   Acute post-infectious glomerulonephritis
B   Amyloidosis
C   Focal and segmental glomerulosclerosis
D   Goodpasture's syndrome
E   IgA nephropathy
F   Light chain disease
G   Membranous nephropathy
H   Mesangiocapillary glomerulonephritis
I   Minimal change glomerulonephritis
J   Systemic lupus erythematosus

1.   A 15-year-old boy presents with swelling of the face and legs. His blood pressure is 195/100 mmHg and the urine appears cloudy and tinged with blood. He is admitted to hospital and treated with a diuretic. He improves so that after 2 weeks he is back to his normal self, with normal renal function. His ASO titre is elevated.

2.   A 46-year-old man presents with swelling of his lower limbs and scrotum. Urinalysis shows heavy proteinuria but no blood or ketones and microscopy is normal. He gives a history of jaundice and is found to be hepatitis B surface antigen positive. His renal function progressively deteriorates and he goes on to have a renal biopsy that shows a thickened basement membrane and granular subepithelial deposits of IgG.

3.   A 19-year-old woman presents with swelling of her legs. She has previously been fit and well. Her blood pressure is normal but urinalysis shows protein +++, ketones +, glucose – and blood –. A renal biopsy is performed and is reported as normal.

4.   A 29-year-old man is known to be HIV positive and presents with generalized oedema. Urinalysis confirms proteinuria and his plasma urea and electrolytes continue to deteriorate. A renal biopsy shows scarring of some glomeruli and scattered immune deposits.

5.   A 60-year-old man presents with haemoptysis and haematuria. His renal function deteriorates rapidly. A renal biopsy shows crescent formation and linear IgG deposits along the basement membrane.

Answers to 6.5

1. **A. Acute post-infectious glomerulonephritis.** The elevated ASO titre suggests a recent infection with a streptococcal strain. Some streptococci induce a glomerulonephritis that presents with oedema, proteinuria, hypertension and haematuria (i.e. the nephrotic syndrome). This usually resolves spontaneously.

2. **G. Membranous nephropathy.** This is the most common cause of nephrotic syndrome in adults. Hepatitis B infection is associated with both membranous nephropathy and mesangiocapillary glomerulonephritis. The subepithelial deposits of IgG and thickened basement membrane are typical of membranous nephropathy—subendothelial deposits are seen in mesangiocapillary nephritis.

3. **I. Minimal change glomerulonephritis.** This accounts for around 25% of adult patients with nephrotic syndrome. Electron microscopy of the renal biopsy reveals fusion of the podocyte foot processes but this is a non-specific finding. The nephrotic syndrome responds to systemic steroids.

4. **C. Focal and segmental glomerulosclerosis.** This form of glomerulonephritis has been reported in several patients with HIV disease. IgA nephropathy is also seen in patients with HIV.

5. **D. Goodpasture's syndrome.** The patient has both pulmonary and renal haemorrhage although both may occur in isolation. Crescent formation is a poor prognostic sign suggesting severe glomerular damage. IgG lines the basement membrane and autoimmunity against the $\alpha 3$ chain of type IV collagen has been reported.

RENAL FAILURE

6.6 Match the most likely diagnosis against each of the following clinical scenarios.

A   Acute interstitial nephritis
B   Acute tubular necrosis
C   Adult polycystic kidney disease
D   Analgesic nephropathy
E   Crystal nephropathy
F   Hepato-renal syndrome
G   Nephrotic syndrome
H   Reflux nephropathy
I   Renal tubular acidosis
J   Sickle-cell nephropathy

1. A 22-year-old Russian journalist has been unable to continue his job because of swelling of his legs and tiredness. On examination, there is oedema of his legs and the genitalia. He has gross proteinuria (urinary albumin 4 g/day) and the serum albumin is 30 g/L.

2. An 8-year-old French boy was collecting the cuttings while his mother was pruning roses. Within 48 h he became toxaemic with a temperature of 39°C and was admitted to hospital. His pulse was 120 bpm and the systolic BP was 90 mmHg. He had failed to produce any urine for the last 12 h.

3. A 30-year-old Welsh singer was diagnosed as having a urinary tract infection and given ampicillin. A few hours after the first dose she developed a blotchy rash and a fever. On admission to hospital, she was found to have eosinophilia, a blood urea of 30 mmol/L and creatinine of 300 mmol/L. Her urine contained a mixture of red blood cells, polymorphs and eosinophils.

4. A 38-year-old nurse of African origin had a long history of backache. She presented with a 3-week history of malaise, thirst and polyuria. She has had colicky abdominal pains in the last 24 h. Both her urea and creatinine are raised. Her blood pressure is 180/110 mmHg. Her urine contains red cell casts and necrotic papillae.

5. A 30-year-old Greek housewife presents with polyuria and polydipsia. In the past, she has had several episodes of severe pain in her chest, abdomen and legs, and was admitted twice with suspected acute cholecystitis. The blood results reveal uraemia and her urine contains necrotic papillae.

Answers to 6.6

1. **G. Nephrotic syndrome.** The description given is typical of nephrotic syndrome with oedema, low serum albumin and a urinary albumin excretion of more than 3.5 g/L. Massive losses of protein lead to other abnormalities which are associated with nephrotic syndrome. These patients tend to have hypercholesterolaemia, a tendency to hypercoagulability and thromboembolism, due to loss of inhibitors of coagulation. A loss of gamma globulins makes them prone to repeated infections.

2. **B. Acute tubular necrosis.** Septicaemia and ensuing dehydration caused vascular collapse and acute tubular necrosis in this young boy, who probably got infected through a rose thorn. These patients rapidly develop uraemia, hyperkalaemia and metabolic acidosis.

3. **A. Acute interstitial nephritis.** About one-third of the cases of interstitial nephritis are caused by a drug in susceptible subjects. The onset is usually abrupt and the presence of eosinophils in the urine is highly suggestive of a hypersensitive reaction. A renal biopsy will be required to establish the diagnosis.

4. **D. Analgesic nephropathy.** This has become increasingly common with the indiscriminate use and over-the-counter availability of analgesic drugs. Chronic ingestion of analgesic drugs causes renal tubular damage and loss of concentrating ability. Renal colic is caused by the passage of necrotic papillary fragments. Asymptomatic patients with uraemia may be picked up at routine medical examination.

5. **J. Sickle-cell nephropathy.** The Mediterranean origin of this patient and a history of cholecystitis and painful crises are important pointers to the diagnosis. Sickle-cell anaemia occurs predominantly in the equatorial Africa and Mediterranean regions. Loss of urinary concentrating ability and polyuria are common in early stages. As in analgesic nephropathy, papillary necrosis is common.

DISORDERS OF THE MALE GENITALIA

6.7 **For each of the following males with a disorder of the male genitalia, select the most likely diagnosis.**

A Balanitis
B Carcinoma of the penis
C Epispadias
D Erectile dysfunction
E Hypospadias
F Non-retractile prepuce
G Paraphimosis
H Peyronie's disease
I Phimosis
J Urethral stricture

1. The mother of a 12-month-old boy seeks advice because she is concerned that she cannot pull back his foreskin when giving him a bath.

2. The mother of a 6-year-old boy seeks advice because she has noticed that the foreskin 'balloons-up' when he passes urine.

3. A 15-year-old boy attends the A&E complaining of pain in his penis. On examination, the glans is swollen and dark blue in colour and appears constricted by a tight band of skin with associated skin oedema.

4. At a routine neonatal check, the urethra of a male child is found to open not at the tip of the penis but midway down the dorsal aspect of the shaft.

5. A 19-year-old man with type 1 diabetes complains of pain on attempting sexual intercourse. On examination, the glans penis is red and inflamed and, although the foreskin retracts fully, there are multiple painful fissures of the skin.

Answers to 6.7

1. **F. Non-retractile prepuce.** This is a normal finding and the parents should be advised not to try to retract the foreskin until the child is at least 3 years old.

2. **I. Phimosis.** This is due to narrowing of the preputial orifice. Circumcision is required.

3. **G. Paraphimosis.** The foreskin has been retracted over the glans (when bathing or during an erection), but it then becomes a constricting, tight band that interferes with venous return from the glans that swells.

4. **C. Epispadias.** This is less common than hypospadias, where the urethra opens on the ventral surface of the penis. *Note* that the terms ventral and dorsal apply to the penis in its 'anatomical', i.e. erect, position.

5. **A. Balanitis.** Inflammation of the glans and foreskin with *Candida* is relatively common in patients with diabetes.

Endocrine system

7.1 The following patients with diabetes are all injecting themselves twice a day with insulin. Select the most logical change to their medication given the scenarios listed below.

A   Change from human to animal derived insulin
B   Decrease long acting insulin in evening
C   Decrease long acting insulin in morning
D   Decrease rapid acting insulin in evening
E   Decrease rapid acting insulin in morning
F   Increase long acting insulin in evening
G   Increase long acting insulin in morning
H   Increase rapid acting insulin in evening
I   Increase rapid acting insulin in morning
J   Withhold insulin for 24 h

1. A patient has consistent and recurrent hypoglycaemia at around 9 p.m.

2. A patient has consistent and recurrent hypoglycaemia in the early hours of the morning.

3. A patient records blood sugars of >14 mmol/L each morning and around 10 mmol/L before going to bed.

4. A patient records blood sugars of >14 mmol/L before lunch on most days.

5. A patient suffers from regular and recurrent hypoglycaemia at around 10 a.m.

Answers to 7.1

1. **D. Decrease rapid acting insulin in evening.** Traditional 'rapid acting' insulin preparations take around 30 min to start working after a subcutaneous injection and last 6–8 h. Hypoglycaemia in the evening can often be prevented by reducing the dose of this type of insulin, especially if the evening meal is going to be light. Newer, genetically modified insulins have a more rapid onset of action.

2. **B. Decrease long acting insulin in the evening.** Insulin preparations such as Monotard or Humulin I will have a significant effect for 10–14 h. Hypoglycaemia in the early hours may be managed by reducing the dose of this type of insulin in the evening. Alternatively, patients may be asked to check blood glucose before going to bed and to eat a snack if the value is low. In general, it is better to reduce the insulin dose, since excessive snacking may lead to undesirable weight gain.

3. **F. Increase long acting insulin in the evening.** In this case, the patient requires more long acting insulin in the evening to help reduce the following morning's blood sugar. The bed-time value of 10 mmol/L is important to note since it suggests that the dose can be increased without precipitating hypoglycaemia earlier in the night.

4. **I. Increase rapid acting insulin in the morning.** Generally the problem here is one of insufficient rapid acting insulin since most people in the UK take their morning insulin and breakfast between 7 a.m. and 8 a.m. (i.e. 4–6 h before lunch). Patients who rise early (e.g. delivery workers) and take their morning insulin before 6 a.m. may need to increase their long acting insulin in the morning or take a mid-morning snack (the most common solution).

5. **E. Decrease rapid acting insulin in the morning.** Around 10 a.m. is a common time for hypoglycaemia if excessive rapid acting insulin has been administered or a patient has left home without an adequate breakfast.

CLASSIFICATION OF DIABETES MELLITUS

7.2 **For each of the following patients with diabetes, select the correct classification.**

A   Diabetes due to chronic pancreatitis
B   Drug induced diabetes
C   Gestational diabetes
D   Haemochromatosis
E   Impaired fasting glycaemia
F   Impaired glucose tolerance
G   Mitochondrial diabetes
H   MODY syndrome
I   Type 1 diabetes
J   Type 2 diabetes

1.   An 84-year-old woman is admitted with weight loss, polyuria and polydipsia. A random blood glucose is 18.4 mmol/L. Islet-cell antibodies and anti-GAD antibodies are present in high titre.

2.   A 15-year-old boy is found to have a random blood glucose of 12 mmol/L. He has no symptoms, is of normal body weight and appears well. Islet-cell antibodies and anti-GAD antibodies are negative. Urinalysis shows glucose ++, ketones –, protein –. His father and paternal grandfather both have diabetes.

3.   A 23-year-old woman with cystic fibrosis has a random blood glucose of 18 mmol/L.

4.   A 60-year-old woman asks to be tested for diabetes because she has polyuria. Her fasting blood glucose is 6.8 mmol/L and, 2 h after a 75 g oral glucose load, the glucose rises to 8.4 mmol/L.

5.   A 52-year-old woman is referred to the diabetes clinic because her glycaemic control is poor. She is not overweight but suffers from bilateral deafness. Her mother and maternal grandmother also have diabetes and deafness. Fundoscopy reveals background diabetic retinopathy and pigmented lesions scattered throughout the fundus.

Answers to 7.2

1. **I. Type 1 diabetes.** Type 1 diabetes may present at any age. The patient has high levels of auto-antibodies associated with islet-cell destruction.

2. **H. MODY syndrome.** Maturity onset diabetes of the young represents a distinct sub-type of diabetes. It is characterized by autosomal dominant inheritance, onset in teenage or early adult life and lack of ketonaemia. A number of mutations in glucokinase and transcription factor genes have been identified in affected families.

3. **A. Diabetes due to chronic pancreatitis.** With improvements in the management of chest problems, more patients with cystic fibrosis are reaching adult life but have a high prevalence of diabetes due to the chronic pancreatic damage caused by the disorder.

4. **E. Impaired fasting glycaemia.** The World Health Organization criteria for the diagnosis of diabetes are a fasting glucose of ≥ 7.0 mmol/L and a glucose of ≥ 11.1 mmol/L after a standard oral glucose load. However, it is recognized that people with a fasting glucose higher than 6.1 mmol/L are not entirely normal (they may be at increased risk of diabetes or macrovascular disease) and so the term impaired fasting glycaemia has been adopted.

5. **G. Mitochondrial diabetes.** There are several diabetes and deafness syndromes, including DIDMOAD (diabetes insipidus, diabetes mellitus, optic atrophy and deafness). The maternal history and pigmented retinopathy are features of mitochondrial diabetes due to mutations in the maternally inherited mitochondrial DNA.

DIABETES AND NEUROPATHY

7.3 **For each of the following patients with neurological complications of diabetes, select the correct diagnosis.**

A   Autonomic neuropathy
B   Cerebrovascular disease
C   Charcot's joint
D   Chronic sensory neuropathy
E   Compression neuropathy
F   Diffuse motor neuropathy
G   Encephalopathy
H   Mononeuritis
I   Proximal motor neuropathy
J   Treatment induced neuropathy

1.   A 61-year-old man with type 2 diabetes presents with an infected ulcer on his right foot. On examination, he has bilateral absent ankle jerks and reduced sensation in all modalities in both legs to the mid-calves.

2.   A 68-year-old woman with type 1 diabetes complains of numbness and tingling in both hands. On examination, she has wasting of both thenar eminences.

3.   A 44-year-old woman with type 1 diabetes presents with diplopia. On examination, the right eye is deviated laterally and inferiorly but the pupil is normal.

4.   A 72-year-old man with type 2 diabetes develops a painful, red, swollen foot. The foot looks infected but there is no ulcer. The foot rapidly becomes deformed.

5.   An 89-year-old man with type 2 diabetes presents with fasciculation in the muscles of both hands and both thighs and increasing muscle weakness. He has diminished ankle jerks but no other sensory signs.

Answers to 7.3

1. **D. Chronic sensory neuropathy.** This is the most common form of neuropathy found in patients with diabetes and predisposes to foot ulceration ('neuropathic ulcer').

2. **E. Compression neuropathy.** The patient has symptoms and signs of bilateral carpal tunnel syndrome. The median nerves are compressed under the flexor retinaculum. Other compression neuropathies such as common peroneal nerve palsies are also more common in patients with diabetes than in the general population.

3. **H. Mononeuritis.** The patient has a single nerve lesion. The IIIrd cranial nerve is relatively commonly affected in diabetes but other single nerves may also be involved as part of a mononeuritis multiplex. Ischaemia is thought to play a major part in the pathogenesis; the pupil is often spared since the parasympathetic fibres are carried on the outside of the nerve and infarction occurs in the core. Compressive lesions, such as an intracranial aneurysm, lead to complete IIIrd nerve palsies, with a dilated pupil.

4. **C. Charcot's joint.** The pathogenesis of this disorder remains far from clear. There is an autonomic component but, in addition, there is rapid osteoporosis of the foot bones, leading to fractures and deformity that sometimes occurs in a matter of days. The increased superficial blood flow makes the foot red and hot.

5. **F. Diffuse motor neuropathy.** This is due to widespread denervation of muscle. Clinically it may be difficult to distinguish from motor neurone disease.

MANAGEMENT OF DIABETES

7.4 **For each of the following patients with diabetes, select the most appropriate treatment.**

A   Commence on insulin
B   Commence on metformin
C   Commence on sulphonylurea
D   Give intramuscular glucagon
E   Give intravenous dextrose
F   Omit metformin
G   Omit morning insulin doses
H   Use rosiglitazone and metformin in combination
I   Use sulphonylurea and metformin in combination
J   Withhold oral hypoglycaemic agents

1. A 30-year-old woman who has been previously fit and well is found to have blood sugars of between 10 and 12 during the first trimester of pregnancy.

2. A 26-year-old woman with type 1 diabetes tried to control her blood glucose very tightly. She had had frequent hypoglycaemic episodes at home but is taken to A&E after collapsing in the street with another attack.

3. A 62-year-old man weighing 90 kg is found to have a random blood sugar of 14.0 mmol/L at a 'Well Man' clinic check-up.

4. A 58-year-old woman has long-standing type 2 diabetes with poor glycaemic control. She has recently been started on insulin but has had several hypoglycaemic episodes. Her husband is concerned that, during the last attack, she was not well enough to swallow any sweet substances.

5. A 70-year-old man with type 2 diabetes has been treated with maximum doses of metformin. However, his blood sugar remains unacceptably high. Apart from metformin, he is on furosemide (frusemide) and an angiotensin-converting enzyme inhibitor for heart failure.

Answers to 7.4

1. **A. Commence on insulin.** The blood sugar is too high but oral hypoglycaemics are not used during pregnancy.

2. **E. Give intravenous dextrose.** Dextrose should be given to any patient with diabetes who has collapsed. Ideally, the blood glucose should be checked beforehand but this must not delay the administration. Glucagon is unlikely to work well in this situation since the recurrent hypoglycaemic episodes will have depleted the liver of glycogen reserves.

3. **J. Withhold oral hypoglycaemic agent.** Diet (low refined carbohydrate and fat) and exercise are the first-line therapy for patients with diabetes.

4. **D. Give intramuscular glucagon.** Relatives of people with diabetes may be shown how to use glucagon. It is available in a kit containing a syringe and needle but needs to be kept in the fridge.

5. **I. Use sulphonylurea and metformin in combination.** Most physicians would add a sulphonylurea at this stage. Rosiglitazone is contraindicated because of the history of heart failure. It would also be acceptable to convert the patient to insulin.

FAMILIAL ENDOCRINE DISORDERS

7.5 **Select the most appropriate diagnosis for each of the following patients.**

A   Autoimmune polyglandular syndrome type 1
B   Autoimmune polyglandular syndrome type 2
C   Familial hypocalciuric hypercalcaemia
D   Hyperparathyroidism
E   Hypoparathyroidism
F   Multiple endocrine neoplasia (MEN) type I
G   Multiple endocrine neoplasia type IIa
H   Multiple endocrine neoplasia type IIb
I   MODY syndrome
J   Pseudohypoparathyroidism

1. A 12-year-old boy is found to have a fasting blood sugar of 8.0 mmol/L. His father and paternal grandfather also have diabetes.

2. A 57-year-old man is found to have an elevated serum calcium as part of a routine biochemical profile. His 24-h urinary calcium is low.

3. A patient is found to have Addison's disease and hypothyroidism.

4. A patient with hypertension is found to have raised levels of urinary adrenaline and noradrenaline. Further investigations show that she has medullary carcinoma of the thyroid.

5. A patient is found to have a low serum calcium, high phosphate and low parathyroid hormone level but thyroid function tests are normal. Her mother has primary hypothyroidism.

Answers to 7.5

1. **I. MODY syndrome.** Maturity onset diabetes of the young is an autosomal dominant disorder. There is insufficient insulin secretion due to a genetic β-cell defect but, since at least some insulin is secreted, ketosis is not a feature.

2. **C. Familial hypocalciuric hypercalcaemia.** Common causes of hypercalcaemia include malignancy and primary hyperparathyroidism. In these conditions, urinary calcium excretion is raised (leading to the risk of renal stones). A low urinary calcium suggests the condition of familial hypocalciuric hypercalcaemia. This is due to mutations in the calcium-sensing receptor gene. It is an important diagnosis to make since affected patients do not benefit from parathyroidectomy even if the serum calcium and PTH are raised.

3. **B. Autoimmune polyglandular syndrome type 2.** This syndrome encompasses Addison's disease, hypothyroidism, hypogonadism, type 1 diabetes, vitiligo and pernicious anaemia. Autoimmune polyglandular syndrome type 1 is characterized by Addison's disease, hypoparathyroidism and chronic mucocutaneous candidiasis.

4. **G. Multiple endocrine neoplasia type IIa.** This is also termed Sipple's syndrome. The patient has a phaeochromocytoma and medullary carcinoma of the thyroid. The other feature of the syndrome is primary hyperparathyroidism. The presence of mucosal neuromata, abnormal dental enamel and Marfanoid features would suggest MEN type IIb. MEN type 1 (Wermer's syndrome) is characterized by primary hyperparathyroidism, functioning pituitary tumours and pancreatic tumours. MEN syndromes are autosomal dominant conditions and should be considered in any patient with two or more endocrine disorders (e.g. hypercalcaemia and a pituitary or pancreatic tumour) and those with a single endocrine abnormality but who also have a family history of endocrine tumours.

5. **E. Hypoparathyroidism.** Common causes include autoimmune destruction (there may be a family history of other autoimmune disease) and post-neck surgery.

ENDOCRINE TESTS

7.6 **For each of the following clinical scenarios, select the most appropriate investigation.**

A   2-h glucose tolerance test
B   Dexamethasone suppression test
C   Domperidone test
D   Insulin-like growth factor 1 (IGF1) measurement
E   Insulin stress test
F   Prolonged fast
G   Prolonged glucose tolerance test
H   Synacthen test
I   TRH test
J   Water deprivation test

1.   A 60-year-old man was found to have acromegaly 8 years ago and underwent a hypophysectomy. He now complains that his hands and feet are swelling and he is beginning to feel like he was before he had his surgery.

2.   A 39-year-old woman complains of recurrent attacks of fainting. She says they usually occur when she has missed a meal.

3.   A 46-year-old man visits his general practitioner complaining of tiredness and lethargy. On examination, he has deeply pigmented skin and oral mucosa.

4.   An 18-year-old man is referred for endocrine assessment following irradiation of a pituitary tumour the previous year. He complains of tiredness, lethargy, weight gain and loss of libido.

5.   A 50-year-old woman is referred to the endocrine clinic with diabetes, hypertension, frontal balding and hirsutism.

Answers to 7.6

1. **D. Insulin-like growth factor 1 measurement.** This history suggests recurrence of the acromegaly. Many patients will have radiotherapy following hypophysectomy to reduce the risk of recurrence. A raised IGF1 level will confirm the diagnosis since excess growth hormone secretion leads to a rise in IGF1.

2. **F. Prolonged fast.** Most patients who are investigated for suspected hypoglycaemic episodes are not found to have a serious endocrine cause for their symptoms. However, the only way of excluding an insulinoma is to perform a well-supervised prolonged fast with blood samples taken for plasma glucose and C-peptide estimations should symptoms occur. A portable glucose meter (e.g. Glucometer®) result is not sufficient and the fast should not be stopped prematurely unless the laboratory assayed plasma glucose is reported as unequivocally low.

3. **H. Synacthen test.** The history suggests Addison's disease, due to destruction of the adrenal glands. A baseline cortisol level will be low with a raised ACTH. Administration of exogenous ACTH (i.e. synacthen) will fail to produce a rise in serum cortisol.

4. **E. Insulin stress test.** Fewer insulin stress tests are being performed because of concerns about safety; they should not be performed in patients with heart disease or a history of epilepsy. Nevertheless, the test remains valuable in the assessment of patients with suspected hypopituitarism. The co-administration of LHRH and TRH allows the combined testing of most parts of the anterior pituitary gland. Increasingly, some authorities rely on a synacthen test to assess the hypothalamo-hypophyseal-adrenal axis. This would be acceptable in this patient providing other tests were performed (e.g. baseline LH, FSH, testosterone and thyroid function tests).

5. **B. Dexamethasone suppression test.** Cushing's disease or syndrome is a possibility given the diabetes, hypertension and hirsutism. Failure of exogenous steroid to suppress adrenal synthesis of glucocorticoids would lend further support to the diagnosis.

MANAGEMENT OF THYROID DISEASE

7.7   **For each of the following clinical scenarios select the most appropriate intervention.**

Normal values: T_4 = 10–27 pmol/L, TSH = 0.15–5.5 mU/L.

A   Give Lugol's iodine
B   Give radio-active iodine
C   No thyroid treatment required
D   Perform fine-needle aspiration of the thyroid
E   Perform thyroidectomy
F   Start carbimazole
G   Start propranolol
H   Start systemic steroids
I   Start thyroxine
J   Stop carbimazole

1.   A 42-year-old woman presents complaining of tiredness, lethargy and weight gain. The T_4 is 10 pmol/L and the TSH is 0.3 mU/L. Examination of the neck is normal.

2.   A 70-year-old woman presents complaining of weight loss, diarrhoea and anxiety. The T_4 is 42 pmol/L and the TSH is <0.01 mU/L. Examination of the neck is normal.

3.   A 50-year-old man complains of severe pain and neck tenderness radiating to the ears, worse on swallowing. The T_4 is 26 pmol/L, TSH 0.1 mU/L, ESR 98. Examination of the neck reveals a tender, smooth goitre but a radioiodine scan shows little uptake.

4.   A 47-year-old woman presents with discomfort in her neck and weight loss. The T_4 is 12 pmol/L and the TSH is 0.2 mU/L. Examination of the neck reveals an irregular-feeling goitre and a radioiodine uptake scan shows a 'cold' nodule.

5.   A 20-year-old woman presents in the first trimester of pregnancy complaining of tiredness and lethargy. The T_4 is 4 pmol/L and the TSH is 26 mU/L. Examination of the neck is normal.

Answers to 7.7

1. **C. No thyroid treatment required.** The patient has normal thyroid function tests. There are many other causes of tiredness, lethargy and weight gain and these should be excluded.

2. **F. Start carbimazole.** The patient has clinical and biochemical features of thyrotoxicosis. The history does not suggest urgency in rendering the patient euthyroid and therefore there is no need to use steroids or Lugol's iodine. Surgery or radiotherapy may be the best long-term treatment, but initially the patient should be treated medically. Propranolol may be used to treat tremor but we are not told that this is a particular problem in this patient. Carbimazole is the most appropriate therapy, although patients need to be warned of the possible adverse reactions (including agranulocytosis).

3. **H. Start systemic steroids.** The history is of De Quervain's thyroiditis. The thyroid function tests may be normal, show thyrotoxicosis or hypothyroidism. The iodine uptake is low because the damaged follicular cells do not trap iodine. The systemic upset and pain may respond to simple analgesics but may be severe enough to require systemic steroid therapy.

4. **D. Perform fine-needle aspiration of the thyroid.** The patient is clinically euthyroid and examination of the neck suggests a multinodular goitre or malignancy (or both, since malignancy may arise in a multinodular goitre). The uptake scan shows a cold nodule. Hot nodules, usually but not always, are benign but cold nodules may or may not be malignant. Surgery may be required but most endocrinologists would initially perform a fine-needle aspiration of the nodule.

5. **I. Start thyroxine.** The patient has primary hypothyroidism. This is a relatively unusual diagnosis in pregnancy, since women with hypothyroidism frequently have irregular periods and relative infertility.

ENDOCRINOLOGY OF SEXUAL DEVELOPMENT AND FUNCTION

7.8 **For each of the following cases, select the most likely diagnosis.**

A Androgen-secreting ovarian tumour
B Congenital adrenal hyperplasia
C Kallmann's syndrome
D Klinefelter's syndrome
E Normal
F Polycystic ovarian syndrome
G Premature ovarian failure
H Testicular feminization syndrome
I Turner's syndrome
J XYY karyotype

1. The parents of a 9-year-old girl attend their general practitioner because they have noticed she has early breast development.

2. A 40-year-old woman is seen in the gynaecology clinic with a 6-month history of irregular periods and hirsutism. On examination, she has signs of virilization.

3. An 18-year-old man is referred to the endocrine clinic by his general practitioner because of delayed pubertal development. As a child, he had a cleft palate repair. On examination, he has poor development of secondary sexual characteristics and his testes are both small and soft.

4. A 40-year-old woman is seen in the gynaecology clinic complaining of irregular, heavy periods and hirsutism. On examination, she is overweight and has acanthosis nigricans in both axillae.

5. A 27-year-old man attends the infertility clinic with his wife. On examination, he is tall and well androgenized. However, he does give a history of delayed puberty, and on examination he has gynaecomastia and bilateral small and hard testes.

Answers to 7.8

1.   **E. Normal.** Thelarche (breast development) is often the first sign of puberty in girls and 9 years of age is not unduly premature.

2.   **A. Androgen-secreting ovarian tumour.** Hirsutism is a very common complaint and in the vast majority of cases no sinister endocrine cause is found. Hirsutism and irregular periods are frequently due to polycystic ovarian syndrome. Virilization (e.g. clitoral hypertrophy) is a much more worrying feature and suggests an underlying androgen-secreting tumour.

3.   **C. Kallmann's syndrome.** This is due to GnRH deficiency. There is failure to develop secondary sexual characteristics and the testes are small and feel soft. Lack of sense of smell and a variety of structural defects (e.g. cleft palate, dextrocardia and urinary tract abnormalities) are associated with the disorder.

4.   **E. Polycystic ovarian syndrome (PCOS).** Insulin resistance is a feature of PCOS and, in severe cases, this is associated with a velvety-thickening of the skin termed acanthosis nigricans.

5.   **D. Klinefelter's syndrome.** This is due to the XXY karyotype. The phenotype can be quite variable with some patients having a near normal puberty, penile size and pubic hair distribution. This results in a few cases not being diagnosed until relatively late. However, the testes are characteristically small and hard and the man is infertile.

THYROID AND PARATHYROID SURGERY

7.9 **Select the most likely diagnosis for each of the following patients with a lump in the neck.**

A Anaplastic carcinoma
B Follicular carcinoma
C Graves' disease
D Haemorrhage into thyroid nodule
E Medullary carcinoma
F Papillary carcinoma
G Parathyroid adenoma
H Parathyroid carcinoma
I Single toxic nodule
J Toxic multinodular goitre

1. A 60-year-old woman is found to be hypercalcaemic with a raised parathyroid hormone concentration. On examination, she has a 1×2 cm lump at the level of the lower lobe of the thyroid gland. The lump is smooth, firm and non-tender.

2. A 22-year-old man is found to be thyrotoxic. On examination, the left lobe of the thyroid is enlarged, smooth and 'fleshy'. The right lobe can just be felt and there is no bruit. He also complains of diplopia and has bilateral exophthalmos.

3. A 19-year-old woman is found to have several lumps in the neck. A biopsy is taken of one of them and the histological appearances are those of well-differentiated thyroid tissue.

4. A 55-year-old woman is seen in the out-patient clinic complaining of a lump in the neck. She is clinically and biochemically euthyroid but an ultrasound scan confirms the lump is lying in the thyroid gland. A fine-needle aspiration is performed and the lump shrinks in size. However, the patient returns the following week complaining that the lump has increased in size again and has become tender.

5. An 80-year-old man complains of a lump in the neck and difficulty in swallowing. On examination, the patient is clinically euthyroid but has a 4×3 cm mass in the anterior triangle of the neck and several smaller lumps in the posterior triangle of the neck. When he attends for an ultrasound scan the following week, he comments that his voice has become hoarse.

Answers to 7.9

1. **G. Parathyroid adenoma.** The two main causes of hypercalcaemia are primary hyperparathyroidism and malignancy. Thyroid disease (malignant or benign) is an exceedingly uncommon cause of a raised serum calcium. Parathyroid carcinoma is rare and usually undifferentiated so that it cannot produce functioning parathyroid (PTH) hormone. Although an adenoma cannot be felt in the neck of most patients with primary hyperparathyroidism, this is still the most likely diagnosis in this woman.

2. **C. Graves' disease.** Exophthalmos is a hallmark of Graves' disease and will not occur in patients with single or multiple toxic nodules. A bruit is heard only in a minority of cases and asymmetrical enlargement of the thyroid is also well recognized.

3. **F. Papillary carcinoma.** The term 'lateral aberrant thyroid' was previously used to describe well-differentiated thyroid tissue occurring outside the thyroid gland in the neck. It is now appreciated that these lesions represent metastatic thyroid cancer in cervical lymph nodes.

4. **D. Haemorrhage into thyroid nodule.** Lumps in the thyroid are a common clinical scenario. Shrinkage after fine-needle aspiration implies that the lump was a fluid-containing follicle. Bleeding may occur, causing the lump to recur or become even larger than originally.

5. **A. Anaplastic carcinoma.** Dysphagia and dysphonia are sinister signs and, in a man of this age, an anaplastic thyroid carcinoma is the most likely of the options listed.

Clinical biochemistry

AUTO-ANTIBODIES IN DISEASE

8.1 **For each of the diseases given below, select the most characteristic auto-antibody that is found in the serum.**

A   Anti-centromere antibodies
B   Anti-glutamic acid decarboxylase antibodies
C   Anti-histone antibodies
D   Anti-Jo-1 antibodies
E   Anti-microsomal antibodies
F   Anti-mitochondrial antibodies
G   Anti-neutrophil cytoplasmic antibodies (pANCA and/or cANCA)
H   Anti-phospholipid antibodies
I   Anti-smooth muscle antibodies
J   TSH receptor antibodies

1.   A patient with type 1 diabetes mellitus.

2.   A patient with Graves' disease.

3.   A patient with Wegener's granulomatosis.

4.   A patient with CREST syndrome.

5.   A patient with drug-induced systemic lupus erythematosus (SLE).

Answers to 8.1

1. **B. Anti-glutamic acid decarboxylase.** Anti-GAD antibodies are also found in the CSF of patients with Stiff Person Syndrome. Other auto-antibodies found in type 1 diabetes include anti-insulin and anti-islet cell antibodies.

2. **J. TSH receptor antibodies.** Antibodies that stimulate the TSH receptors produce thyrotoxicosis in Graves' disease. TSH receptor blocking antibodies may also be present.

3. **G. Anti-neutrophil cytoplasmic antibodies.** These may be of either perinuclear (pANCA) or cytoplasmic (cANCA) configuration.

4. **A. Anti-centromere antibodies.** Ninety per cent of patients with CREST (calcinosis, Raynaud's, oesophageal dysmotility, scleroderma and telangiectasia) have anti-centromere antibodies in their serum.

5. **C. Anti-histone antibodies.** Histones are the proteins that envelop chromosomal DNA in the nucleus on cells.

CEREBROSPINAL FLUID

8.2 **A list of results from cerebrospinal fluid (CSF) analysis is given below. For each of the disease states that follow, select the most characteristic CSF finding (assume that the plasma glucose is 6 mmol/L).**

A Blood-stained fluid, pressure normal, 500 cells/μL (red cells) but reducing in quantity in successive bottles, protein 0.2 g/L, glucose 5 mmol/L

B Clear fluid, increased pressure, 900 cells/μL (90% lymphocytes), protein 0.4 g/L, glucose 4 mmol/L

C Clear fluid, normal pressure, 5 cells/μL (lymphocytes), protein 0.3 g/L, glucose 4 mmol/L

D Clear fluid, raised pressure, 15 cells/μL (small cells with dense nuclei), protein 1 g/L, glucose 2 mmol/L

E Clear fluid, raised pressure, 3 cells/μL (lymphocytes), protein 0.3 g/L, glucose 4 mmol/L

F Cloudy fluid, pressure raised, 280 cells/μL (mixed population), protein 0.7 g/L, glucose 2 mmol/L

G Dry tap. Unable to obtain any fluid

H Purulent fluid, raised pressure, >1000 cells/μL (60% neutrophils), protein 0.9 g/L, glucose 2 mmol/L

I Viscous fluid that clots on standing, raised pressure, 300 cells/μL (80% lymphocytes), protein 4 g/L, glucose undetectable

J Yellow fluid, pressure raised, 200 cells/μL (red cells) with no reduction in successive bottles, protein 0.4 g/L, glucose 4 mmol/L

1. A patient with tuberculous meningitis.

2. A patient with meningococcal meningitis.

3. A patient with cryptococcal meningitis.

4. A patient with a subarachnoid haemorrhage.

5. A patient with malignant infiltration of the CSF.

Answers to 8.2

Answer **C** represents the findings in a normal individual.

1. **I.** The CSF in tuberculous meningitis has a very high protein content, is highly viscous, contains a predominance of lymphocytes and a very low glucose concentration.

2. **H.** Bacterial meningitis is characterized by a purulent CSF with a high neutrophil count. The CSF glucose concentration is less than half of that in the plasma. If bacterial meningitis is suspected, treatment should not be delayed pending the results of a lumbar puncture.

3. **F.** Fungal meningitis may occur in immunocompromised patients such as those on immunosuppressants or with HIV/AIDS. The CSF is cloudy with raised pressure and a mixed population of cells.

4. **J.** A traumatic tap will produce blood-stained CSF but the red blood cell count falls with samples taken in successive tubes. In subarachnoid haemorrhage, the red cell count remains high. If the lumbar puncture is delayed for several hours after the haemorrhage, the red cells lyse, giving the CSF a yellowish tinge termed xanthochromia.

5. **D.** Malignancy may infiltrate the arachnoid mater and neoplastic cells seed themselves through the CSF. Cytological examination of the fluid may reveal small numbers of malignant cells with atypical nuclei. The CSF protein is often raised.

SERUM ENZYMES IN CLINICAL DIAGNOSIS

8.3 **For each of the following scenarios, select the most useful enzyme analysis.**

A α-fetoprotein
B AST
C Bilirubin
D CEA
E CK BB
F CK MB
G CK MM
H LDH
I PSA
J Troponin T

1. A 28-year-old woman with a past history of a hydatidiform mole complains of chest pain, shortness of breath and weight loss.

2. A 58-year-old man with a past history of alcoholic liver disease presents with worsening ascites, a continuous dull ache in the abdomen, anorexia and weight loss.

3. A 30-year-old man with a family history of limb-girdle dystrophy presents with difficulty in raising his arms and tenderness of the shoulder girdle muscles.

4. An 80-year-old man presents with confusion and chest pain. A bone scan reveals several sclerotic lesions in the ribs.

5. A 54-year-old woman presents with a 1-h history of dull central chest pain suspicious of a myocardial infarction. However, her ECG appears normal.

Answers to 8.3

1. **D. CEA.** Carcino-embryonic antigen is secreted by invasive choriocarcinomas.

2. **A. α-fetoprotein.** Deterioration in a patient with cirrhosis should suggest the possible development of a hepatocellular carcinoma.

3. **G. CK MM.** Creatine kinase exists in two main forms (M = Muscle, B = Brain). Somatic muscle damage, as with this patient who shows signs of an inherited myopathy, results in a raised CK MM isoform.

4. **I. PSA.** Prostatic specific antigen is raised in patients with invasive prostatic carcinoma. Metastases are typically osteosclerotic.

5. **J. Troponin T.** Troponin molecules are released within hours of a myocardial infarction and also in unstable angina, even if the ECG is normal. The first ECG is normal in about 25% of patients with acute myocardial infarction.

FLUID AND ELECTROLYTE DISTURBANCES

8.4 **For each of the following clinical scenarios, select the most appropriate description of the fluid and electrolyte situation.**

A   Between 2–4 L of fluid loss
B   Greater than 4 L of fluid loss
C K^+ and water loss
D   Less than 2 L of fluid gain
E   Less than 2 L of fluid loss
F   Metabolic acidosis
G   Metabolic alkalosis
H   More than 4 L of fluid gain
I Na^+ and water loss
J   Pure water loss

1.   An 80-year-old woman is admitted to hospital in a confused state. She has reduced skin turgor and cold, cyanosed extremities. Her blood pressure is 90/60 mmHg.

2.   A 42-year-old man with alcoholic liver disease is found to have developed tense ascites.

3.   A 68-year-old man is seen in the medical out-patient clinic with a 3-week history of profuse diarrhoea. Sigmoidoscopy reveals a sessile tumour in the rectum.

4.   A 40-year-old woman is taking lithium carbonate for bipolar affective disorder. She complains of intense thirst, polyuria and nocturia.

5.   A 26-year-old woman is found to have renal tubular acidosis.

Answers to 8.4

1. **B. Greater than 4 L of fluid loss.** Reduced skin turgor, hypotension and confusion all suggest severe fluid depletion. The limited history given does not allow accurate speculation regarding the nature of the electrolyte loss.

2. **H. More than 4 L of fluid gain.** A patient with tense ascites may have over 10 L of fluid in the abdomen.

3. **C. K^+ and water loss.** Although the patient would have lost Na^+ as well as K^+, this is a classic description of a patient with a villous adenoma, resulting in a potassium-losing diarrhoea. H^+ ions are also lost with the K^+ ions, so the patient may additionally have a metabolic alkalosis. Some villous adenomas secrete excessive mucus with loss of protein causing hypoalbuminaemia.

4. **J. Pure water loss.** Lithium causes a nephrogenic (vasopressin resistant) diabetes insipidus so the patient will lose water. She is unlikely to be significantly dehydrated providing she has free access to water to quench her polydipsia.

5. **F. Metabolic acidosis.** Renal tubular acidosis is characterized by inability to lower the urinary pH. In the proximal variety there is reduced bicarbonate absorption leading to bicarbonate wasting and a metabolic acidosis. In the classic distal variety, there is a hypokalaemic, hyperchloraemic metabolic acidosis due to a selective defect in distal acidification (i.e. reduced activity of Na^+/H^+ exchange leading to H^+ accumulation in the blood).

ELECTROLYTE DISTURBANCES

8.5 Select the most characteristic electrolyte disturbance in the following clinical situations.

A   Hypercalcaemia
B   Hyperkalaemia
C   Hypernatraemia
D   Hyperphosphataemia
E   Hypocalcaemia
F   Hypokalaemia
G   Hypomagnesaemia
H   Hyponatraemia
I   Hypophosphataemia
J   Lactic acidosis

1.   A patient with inappropriate ADH secretion.

2.   A patient with tertiary hyperparathyroidism.

3.   A patient with neuroleptic malignant syndrome.

4.   A patient with Bartter's syndrome.

5.   A patient with MELAS syndrome.

Answers to 8.5

1. **H. Hyponatraemia.** Common causes of this syndrome include chest infections, strokes and drugs (e.g. opiates). The kidneys retain an excess of water, thus diluting the serum sodium. The patient does not look dehydrated and urine osmolality is high despite the low serum osmolality.

2. **A. Hypercalcaemia.** Primary hyperparathyroidism (e.g. due to an adenoma of the parathyroid glands) causes hypercalcaemia. Secondary hyperparathyroidism is the term used to describe a compensatory rise in parathyroid hormone levels, e.g. in chronic renal failure or osteomalacia, where the calcium levels tend to be low. The continued stimulation of the parathyroid glands in chronic renal failure may result in tertiary hyperparathyroidism—the glands become 'autonomous' and continue to secrete excess PTH despite raised serum calcium levels.

3. **D. Hyperphosphataemia.** Massive cell necrosis such as occurs in the neuroleptic syndrome or acute rhabdomyolysis results in a transiently raised serum phosphate level. Sustained hyperphosphataemia occurs in renal insufficiency, hypoparathyroidism and acromegaly.

4. **F. Hypokalaemia.** Bartter's syndrome is caused by a mutation in the gene coding for the Na/K transporter in the loop of Henle or in genes encoding calcium or potassium channels. There is profound Na$^+$ and K$^+$ wasting and compensatory hypertrophy of the juxtaglomerular apparatus with hyper-reninaemia.

5. **J. Lactic acidosis.** Mitochondrial myopathies are due to mutations in the mitochondrial DNA. Abnormal Krebs' cycle metabolism results in the accumulation of lactate (e.g. MELAS syndrome = mitochondrial encephalomyopathy, lactic acidosis and stroke-like episodes).

MANAGEMENT OF FLUID AND ELECTROLYTE LOSS

8.6 **For each of the following patients, select the most appropriate management.**

A   Administer 20% dextrose
B   Administer 5% dextrose
C   Administer a plasma expander (colloid)
D   Administer blood
E   Administer dextrose and insulin
F   Administer intravenous calcium
G   Administer normal saline
H   Administer 100 mL of bicarbonate
I   Administer 5-times normal saline
J   Withhold all fluid replacement

1.   You are asked to review a patient who had a parathyroidectomy for primary hyperparathyroidism earlier in the day. The patient is complaining of pins-and-needles in both hands and face. On examination, she has carpopedal spasm.

2.   You are asked to drain the ascites from a patient with probable alcoholic liver disease. After you finish, the patient complains of feeling unwell and looks grey. His blood pressure is 70/40 mmHg.

3.   You admit a patient who has been vomiting for several days. On examination, he is clearly dehydrated but the blood pressure is normal. You check his plasma electrolytes and they are reported as Na⁺ 115 mmol/L, K⁺ 5.0 mmol/L, urea 12 mmol/L and creatinine 130 mmol/L. The urinary sodium is low.

4.   You are called by the biochemist with the following results: Na⁺ 135 mmol/L, K⁺ 7.5 mmol/L, urea 125 mmol/L, creatinine 1800 mmol/L. You review the patient to whom the results belong and find that he has been admitted earlier in the day complaining of nausea and malaise.

5.   An 84-year-old woman is admitted from her residential home in a comatose state. She is normally quite well and her only regular medication is chlorpropamide. Her blood glucose tested at the bedside is 3.0 mmol/L.

Answers to 8.6

1. **F. Administer intravenous calcium.** The patient is likely to have postoperative hypocalcaemia and is at risk of upper-airways spasm or seizures unless it is corrected without delay.

2. **C. Administer a plasma expander.** It is unwise to drain large volumes of ascites since patients may develop profound hypotension following the procedure and, in any case, the ascites tends to re-accumulate rapidly. Intravenous saline should be avoided in liver disease.

3. **G. Administer normal saline.** The patient has hyponatraemia in the face of dehydration with a history of vomiting. He has lost significant amounts of salt and water and saline is the appropriate fluid to use for replacement. There is no need for colloid since the blood pressure is well maintained. Some authorities advocate the use of high concentrations of sodium (e.g. 5-times normal saline) if the hyponatraemia is acute and associated with profound neurological disturbance. However, rapid correction of the hyponatraemia may be dangerous and the serum Na^+ will usually rise satisfactorily with the use of normal saline.

4. **E. Administer dextrose and insulin.** The patient is in renal failure. The hyperkalaemia is a medical emergency since it may lead to a fatal arrhythmia and should be treated with intravenous dextrose and insulin.

5. **A. Administer 20% dextrose.** The patient may be hypoglycaemic. Chlorpropamide is a sulphonylurea with a long half-life and should be avoided in the elderly. Blood glucose testing strips are not particularly accurate at the lower end of the normal range and a laboratory blood sugar should be checked. However, intravenous glucose should be tried before waiting for the result to return. It is safer to administer 20% dextrose than 50% dextrose since it causes less tissue damage if accidentally extravasated into the tissues. A single bolus administration of dextrose may not be enough as chlorpropamide has a long half-life and tends to cause recurrent hypoglycaemia. The plasma glucose should be tested hourly until a stable normal level has been achieved.

PATHOLOGICAL PROTEIN DEPOSITION

8.7 **For each of the following disorders, select the correct fibril-forming protein that results in abnormal protein deposition within tissues.**

A β_2 microglobulin
B β-amyloid precursor
C Amyloid A protein
D Cystatin C
E Immunoglobulin H chain
F Immunoglobulin L chain
G Islet amyloid polypeptide
H Metalloprotein
I Prion protein
J Transthyretin

1. Type 2 diabetes.

2. Alzheimer's disease.

3. Spongiform encephalopathy.

4. Dialysis associated amyloid.

5. Familial Mediterranean fever.

Answers to 8.7

1. **G. Islet amyloid polypeptide (IAPP).** This protein is co-secreted with insulin from the pancreatic β cell. The pathological hallmark of type 2 diabetes is the accumulation of deposits of amyloid formed by the cross-linking of IAPP.

2. **B. β-amyloid precursor.** Neurofibrillary tangles are composed of this protein.

3. **I. Prion protein.** Spongiform encephalopathies include kuru, Creutzfeldt–Jakob (CJD) disease and new variant CJD and are due to the accumulation of an abnormal prion protein.

4. **A. β_2 microglobulin.** Usually occurs in amyloidosis associated with renal failure and long-term dialysis.

5. **C. Amyloid A protein.** Amyloidosis with renal deposition of amyloid A protein is the main complication of familial Mediterranean fever.

9

Rheumatology and orthopaedics

TREATMENTS IN RHEUMATOLOGY

9.1 Select the condition most likely to benefit from each of the following drug treatments.

A   Ankylosing spondylitis
B   Gout
C   Infected joint
D   Lumbar spondylosis
E   Osteoarthrosis
F   Osteomalacia
G   Paget's disease
H   Pseudogout
I   Rheumatoid arthritis
J   Spondylolisthesis

1.   Calcium and vitamin D.

2.   Intravenous antibiotics.

3.   Allopurinol.

4.   Etidronate.

5.   Systemic steroids.

Answers to 9.1

1. **F. Osteomalacia.** Osteomalacia is caused by vitamin D deficiency. Treatment is with the active forms of vitamin D, e.g. Iα-cholecalciferol.

2. **C. Infected joint.** Septic arthritis requires prompt treatment with antibiotics if septicaemia and joint destruction are to be prevented.

3. **B. Gout.** When used on a long-term basis, allopurinol will reduce serum uric acid levels. However, levels may rise transiently at the beginning of treatment and it may precipitate an acute attack.

4. **G. Paget's disease.** Bisphosphonates have become the treatment of choice in painful Paget's disease.

5. **I. Rheumatoid arthritis.** Some patients require high doses of long-term steroids and adequate osteoporosis prophylaxis should be co-administered.

WRIST INJURIES

9.2 **For each of the following scenarios, select the most likely diagnosis.**

A   Colles' fracture
B   Greenstick fracture
C   Hook of hamate fracture
D   Lunate dislocation
E   Pisiform fracture
F   Scaphoid fracture
G   Slipped distal radial epiphysis
H   Smith's fracture
I   Trans-scapho-perilunar dislocation
J   Triquetral fracture

1.   A 20-year-old man has fallen on his outstretched right hand. Examination reveals tenderness in the anatomical snuff-box. An X-ray of the hand reveals a fracture in one of the carpal bones.

2.   A 7-year-old boy has fallen and injured his right wrist. The X-ray shows a slight buckling in the distal radius.

3.   A 70-year-old woman has fallen on her outstretched left hand. Examination of her left wrist reveals a dinner fork deformity.

4.   A 20-year-old man has fallen in a game of football. An X-ray of the wrist reveals a fracture in the distal end of the radius; the distal fragment is anteriorly displaced.

5.   A 20-year-old man has fallen and injured his right wrist. The only abnormality on the X-ray of the wrist is the 'emptying of the lunate cup'.

Answers to 9.2

1. **F. Scaphoid fracture.** This is a frequently missed fracture because a fracture line may not be evident on the initial X-rays. The patient should be reviewed after about 10 days and the X-ray repeated if there is persistent tenderness in the anatomical snuff-box. Inadequate treatment may result in non-union of the fracture and avascular necrosis, causing significant functional impairment.

2. **B. Greenstick fracture.** Children's bones are springy and can react unpredictably to applied force. An angulation force may bend the cortex on one side and cause a buckling or fracture in the cortex on the opposite side. Hence, the radiological evidence of a greenstick fracture may only be a small, localized area of buckling in the cortex. For this reason, it is a commonly missed fracture.

3. **A. Colles' fracture.** This is a common fracture caused by a fall on an outstretched hand. The distal fragment of the radial fracture is displaced and tilted dorsally and hence the deformity is described as simulating a dinner fork. It occurs more frequently in older patients with osteoporosis.

4. **H. Smith's fracture.** This is the reverse of a Colles' fracture in terms of the opposite direction of displacement and angulation. It is an unstable fracture and its reduction is often difficult to maintain after closed manipulation. Surgery is often necessary.

5. **D. Lunate dislocation.** The capitate bone normally sits on top of the lunate cup. With dislocation of the lunate, the lunate rotates through 90° and comes to lie anteriorly. The median nerve is at risk in such an injury.

HAND INJURIES

9.3 **For each of the following scenarios, select the most likely injury.**

A   Abductor pollicis longus injury
B   Boutonnière deformity
C   Digital artery injury
D   Digital nerve injury
E   Extensor digitorum communis tendon injury
F   Extensor pollicis longus tendon injury
G   Flexor digitorum profundus tendon injury
H   Flexor digitorum superficialis tendon injury
I   Flexor pollicis longus tendon injury
J   Mallet finger

1. Following sustaining a cut to the base of his thumb, the patient is unable to flex his thumb at the interphalangeal joint.

2. A rugby player injures his right ring finger while trying to grab an opponent's jersey. He is unable to flex the distal interphalangeal joint of his finger.

3. A 35-year-old lady, while making a bed, caught her right ring finger on a blanket. She is unable to actively extend her finger at the distal interphalangeal joint.

4. Following an injury to his finger a patient develops a flexion deformity at the proximal interphalangeal joint and hyperextension at the distal interphalangeal joint.

5. A patient falls on broken glass and sustains an incised wound over the dorsum of his right hand. He is able to extend both interphalangeal joints but not the metacarpophalangeal joint of his middle finger.

Answers to 9.3

1. **I. Injury to flexor pollicis longus tendon.** The tendon of the flexor pollicis longus is inserted at the palmar aspect of the base of the terminal phalanx of the thumb. The action of the muscle is flexion of the thumb at the interphalangeal joint.

2. **G. Injury to the flexor digitorum profundus tendon.** This indeed is also called the 'jersey finger injury' and is a common mode of injury, sustained as described in the scenario. It is almost always in the ring finger. Treatment is surgical repair.

3. **J. Mallet finger.** This deformity is caused by forced flexion of a finger in an extended position. The extensor tendon is torn from its attachment at the base of the terminal phalanx. Often there is an associated avulsion fracture. In most cases, treatment is by a splint.

4. **B. Boutonnière deformity.** The reverse of this is called a swan-neck deformity. Boutonnière deformity may be caused by an injury to the middle slip extensor tendon at the dorsal aspect of the proximal interphalangeal joint.

5. **E. Injury to extensor digitorum communis tendon.** Extensor digitorum communis is the sole extensor of the metacarpophalangeal joint. Extension at the interphalangeal joints can be achieved by the action of the lumbricals.

KNEE TRAUMA

9.4 **For each of the following scenarios, select the most likely diagnosis.**

A   Anterior cruciate ligament injury
B   Dislocation of the knee
C   Dislocation of the patella
D   Lateral meniscus injury
E   Medial collateral ligament injury
F   Medial meniscus injury
G   Osgood–Schlatter's disease
H   Osteochondral fracture
I   Patella fracture
J   Posterior cruciate ligament injury

1.   A 25-year-old man injured his right knee in a game of football 6 months ago. There was considerable swelling in his knee at the time of injury. On examination now, the anterior draw sign is positive.

2.   A 17-year-old girl has been having problems with both her knees for some time. The pain is in the front of the knees and is worse on descending stairs. She presents to the A&E department following a twisting injury to her right knee while dancing. She is in a lot of pain, and on examination the knee is deformed with gross restriction in movements.

3.   A 25-year-old man had a twisting injury to his right knee 6 months ago. Since the injury, he has had episodes when his knee suddenly 'gives way'. Examination reveals tenderness over the medial joint line and a positive McMurray's sign.

4.   A 25-year-old skier has a fall. Examination reveals tenderness over the medial femoral condyle. Pain is worse on valgus stress.

5.   A 14-year-old boy, a keen football and rugby player, has been experiencing pain in his right knee, especially following exercise. He cannot recall any injury. Examination reveals a tender bony swelling over the tibial tubercle.

Answers to 9.4

1. **A. Anterior cruciate ligament (ACL) injury.** A positive anterior draw sign (with the semi-flexed knee, the tibia yields when pulled forwards) suggests anterior instability—a classical feature of an ACL-deficient knee. The ACL holds the tibia back in a stable knee joint. The swelling at the time of the injury suggests haemarthrosis, of which acute ACL injury is one of the most common causes.

2. **C. Dislocation of the patella.** Her pre-existing symptoms suggest patellofemoral joint pathology. The patella is displaced laterally and can usually be reduced fairly easily without the need of general anaesthesia.

3. **F. Medial meniscus injury.** McMurray's manoeuvre (with the patient supine, the knee is flexed and the foot is rotated medially and laterally, while bringing the knee to 90° of flexion, causing discomfort or a click in the presence of a tear) is used to detect meniscal injuries though in the acute phase it may be too painful to use. The joint-line tenderness may be the only sign. Meniscal tear is often a result of a twisting injury to a semi-flexed weight-bearing knee.

4. **E. Medial collateral ligament injury.** The medial collateral ligament is proximally attached to the medial femoral condyle. Distally it is attached to the proximal part of the tibia, at a variable distance of up to 10 cm below the medial joint line. It is injured by a valgus force.

5. **G. Osgood–Schlatter's disease.** Osteochondritis of the epiphysis of the tibial tuberosity is a common problem caused by overuse of the knee joints in teenagers who regularly participate in a variety of sports. The tibial tubercle is the point of insertion of the extensor mechanism of the knee through the patellar ligament.

SHOULDER/ARM TRAUMA

9.5 **For each the following scenarios, select the most likely diagnosis.**

A   Acromioclavicular joint dislocation
B   Anterior dislocation of the shoulder
C   Brachial plexus injury
D   Clavicle fracture
E   Greater tuberosity of the humerus fracture
F   Humeral shaft fracture
G   Posterior dislocation of the shoulder
H   Rupture of long head of biceps
I   Scapular fracture
J   Supraspinatus tendinitis

1.   A 45-year-old labourer develops pain in his right shoulder while lifting concrete blocks. Examination reveals a painful abduction arc. An area of calcification adjacent to the head of humerus is seen on the X-ray.

2.   A 40-year-old man injures his right arm in a motorcycle accident. His arm is flail and he needs to support it with his other hand. Clinically, there is also evidence of a radial nerve palsy.

3.   A 20-year-old student injures his left shoulder in a rugby tackle. Examination reveals a bony prominence at the lateral end of his clavicle. The X-ray of the shoulder does not reveal any fracture but confirms a superior displacement of the lateral end of the clavicle.

4.   A 20-year-old student injures his left shoulder in a game of rugby. The shoulder looks deformed with a prominent acromion. There is loss of sensation over the 'regimental badge' area of his corresponding arm.

5.   A 35-year-old man injures his right shoulder during an epileptic fit. An A–P view X-ray of his shoulder reveals the 'light bulb sign'. There is flattening in the front of the shoulder and external rotation is severely restricted.

Answers to 9.5

1.   **J. Supraspinatus tendonitis.** This is a common problem, often resulting from overuse of the shoulder joint. Calcification in the tendon suggests a long-standing problem. There is pain when the tendon impinges beneath the acromion, as the arm is abducted to about 60°. Supraspinatus muscle initiates abduction at the shoulder joint.

2.   **F. Humeral shaft fracture.** The radial nerve runs along the spiral grove of the humerus and can be damaged in humeral shaft fracture. The pain is considerable and the patient can often sense the instability.

3.   **A. Acromioclavicular joint dislocation.** Subluxation, when only the capsule of the acromioclavicular joint is torn, is a common injury. Dislocation occurs when in addition the conoid and trapezoid ligaments are also torn. Most cases are treated conservatively with a sling.

4.   **B. Anterior dislocation of the shoulder.** This injury of the shoulder may involve the axillary nerve, causing paralysis of the deltoid muscle. In the acute phase, it is impossible to assess deltoid function but sensory supply to the 'regimental badge' area (an oval area on the lateral surface in the middle of the arm) is easy to test. The problem can become recurrent and surgical repair may be necessary. In anterior dislocation, the head of the humerus rotates out of the glenohumeral joint and comes to lie under the coracoid process. The acromion process thus becomes prominent.

5.   **G. Posterior dislocation of the shoulder.** The injury can easily be missed if only an A–P X-ray is taken, as it is often normal or may only show the 'light bulb sign' due to internal rotation of the shoulder. Supplementary views, such as the axial and Y views, are vital for the diagnosis. The injury often results from severe muscle spasm, such as can occur during an epileptic fit or electric shock.

ELBOW TRAUMA

9.6 **For each of the following scenarios, select the most likely diagnosis.**

A   Bicipital tendinitis
B   Galeazzi's fracture
C   Lateral epicondylitis
D   Medial epicondylar fracture
E   Medial epicondylitis
F   Monteggia's fracture
G   Olecranon bursitis
H   Olecranon fracture
I   Pulled elbow
J   Radial head fracture

1.   A 20-year-old man falls heavily on his right elbow in a game of rugby. The X-rays reveal dislocation of the radial head and a fracture in the proximal shaft of the ulna.

2.   A 2-year-old boy tries to run across a road, his mother grabs his right hand to pull him back. Since then he has not been able to use his right arm. He is holding his arm with the elbow in slight flexion and forearm in pronation. An X-ray of his elbow is normal.

3.   A 7-year-old boy sustains an abduction injury to his right elbow. There is bruising over the medial aspect of his elbow. The medial epicondyle cannot be seen on the X-ray.

4.   A 30-year-old painter complains of pain over the lateral aspect of his right elbow. There is no history of trauma. Clinically, there is tenderness over the common extensor origin.

5.   A 25-year-old man falls on his outstretched hand and sustains a fracture in his right elbow. There is tenderness over the posterolateral aspect of his elbow, pain is worse on supination and pronation and he is unable to fully extend his elbow.

Answers to 9.6

1. **F. Monteggia's fracture.** This is a description of Monteggia's fracture, so called after a Milanese physician who described a fracture of the shaft of the ulna with dislocation of the head of the radius. The opposite—fracture of the radial shaft with dislocation of the inferior radio-ulna joint—is called Galeazzi's (orthopaedic surgeon also from Milan) fracture.

2. **I. Pulled elbow.** This is caused by a traction injury to the elbow, resulting in the head of the radius slipping out of the annular ligament. Reduction is easily achieved by supination of the arm.

3. **D. Medial epicondylar fracture.** The medial epicondyle epiphysis should appear by the age of 6. In this case, the avulsed fragment has gone into the joint and cannot be seen on the X-ray. Unless the doctor interpreting the X-rays has the knowledge of the timing of the appearance of the various epiphyses, such injury is easily missed.

4. **C. Lateral epicondylitis.** This is the most common overuse problem of the elbow, commonly occurring in tennis players and known as the 'tennis elbow'. The lateral epicondyle is the common extensor origin.

5. **J. Radial head fracture.** This is the most common fracture of the elbow. It can be caused by direct trauma but more commonly, indirectly, through a fall on an outstretched hand. The force of the impact is transmitted up the radius causing a fracture in the radial head.

INVESTIGATION OF A SWOLLEN KNEE JOINT

9.7 For each of these scenarios of a swollen knee joint, match the initial key investigation that is most likely to yield the diagnosis.

A   Angiogram
B   Arthrogram
C   Arthroscopy
D   Aspiration and microscopic examination
E   CT scan
F   Doppler of the leg
G   MRI scan
H   Plain X-ray of the knee joint
I   Serum uric acid levels
J   Venogram of the leg

1. A 70-year-old man with ischaemic heart disease has been admitted with left ventricular failure of recent onset. His cardiac echocardiogram showed an ejection fraction of 25%. The treatment was started with bed rest, oxygen inhalation and furosemide (frusemide). On the third day after his admission, he developed a painful swelling of his right knee joint. He cannot move his knee because of pain and the joint looks swollen, erythematous and is tender to touch.

2. A 74-year-old woman with diabetes mellitus and osteoarthrosis is found to have a swollen, painful left knee joint. She has had osteoarthrosis of the knees before but this time the joint is visibly swollen and the movements are limited because of pain.

3. A 27-year-old housewife is admitted to hospital complaining of pain and swelling around her right knee and calf. She recalls twisting her ankle while rushing to catch a plane in California, 2 days previously.

4. A 37-year-old woman with rheumatoid arthritis suddenly felt a click in her right knee joint while she was walking her dog. She felt pain in her knee and leg and had some difficulty in getting home. Her husband brought her to the A&E where she was found to have swelling of the right knee joint and the calf. Movements at the knee joint were restricted and painful.

5. A professional football player for 18 years finds that his left knee has started to give way unexpectedly during training and there is a risk that he will not be fit to play in the Cup Final in 3 weeks' time. Although he has had several minor injuries in his career, he cannot recall recent serious trauma to his knee.

Answers to 9.7

1. **D. Aspiration and microscopic examination.** The most probable diagnosis is acute gout resulting from hyperuricaemia, precipitated by dehydration induced by furosemide (frusemide). The diagnosis can be made by aspirating the joint and examining the fluid under a microscope with polarized light; the brightly birefringent urate crystals can be seen with negative elongation. Serum uric acid levels are not the investigation of choice since they may be normal and, even if raised, the arthritis could be due to another cause.

2. **H. Plain X-ray of the knee joint.** This patient probably has pseudogout that can occur in elderly patients with a variety of conditions such as diabetes mellitus, hyperparathyroidism, haemochromatosis, myxoedema and hypophosphatasia. It is a form of crystal arthropathy caused by the deposition of calcium pyrophosphate crystals. Diagnosis can be made by taking a plain film of the knee joint to show chondrocalcinosis. The knee joint can be aspirated and the fluid examined under the polarized light for the presence of weakly positive birefringent pyrophosphate crystals.

3. **F. Doppler of the leg.** Swelling of the calf as well as the knee is suspicious of a deep vein thrombosis. This woman had hurt her leg shortly before a long-haul flight and had sat in a cramped seat for over 12 h with little exercise. Although airlines have had much adverse publicity regarding the risk of deep vein thrombosis, any long period of immobility increases the risk, including car, coach and rail travel.

4. **B. Arthrogram.** From the story given, the patient has rheumatoid arthritis, and a sudden appearance of swelling involving the knee joint as well as the upper compartment of the calf muscles. This patient has probably ruptured her popliteal synovial membrane (Baker's cyst). The diagnosis can be made on clinical examination and confirmed by an arthrogram when the dye can be seen entering from the joint into the calf muscles. Sometimes it can be confused with deep venous thrombosis, and the diagnosis can be made non-invasively with Doppler study of the leg veins.

5. **G. MRI scan.** This man may have suffered damage to one of the knee ligaments. Since his livelihood depends on an accurate diagnosis, an MRI scan should be performed. This will give better definition than a CT scan. Arthroscopy may be required but, as it is an invasive procedure, imaging techniques should be used first.

AUTO-ANTIBODIES IN RHEUMATOLOGY

9.8 **For each of the following patients, select the most characteristic auto-antibody profile.**

A   Anti-centromere antibodies
B   Anti-Jo-1
C   Anti-La
D   Anti-ds DNA
E   Anti-histone H1, H3, H4
F   Anti-histone H2a, H2b
G   Anti-mitochondrial antibodies
H   Anti-topoisomerase
I   cANCA
J   pANCA

1. A 58-year-old woman complains of dry eyes and a dry mouth. Schirmer's tear test reveals reduced lacrimal secretion.

2. A 52-year-old woman complains of a several month history of weakness and difficulty in climbing stairs. On examination, she has fissuring of the skin of her hands and a chest X-ray shows pulmonary fibrosis.

3. A 63-year-old woman complains of symptoms suggestive of Raynaud's phenomenon and difficulty in swallowing. On examination, she has painful lesions on the tips of her fingers and facial telangiectasia.

4. A 70-year-old man presents with acute renal failure. He has been troubled for many years by recurrent nose bleeds, but over the last 2 weeks he has also been coughing up blood-stained sputum.

5. A 70-year-old man presents with a Bell's palsy. His medical history includes late onset asthma and heart failure. He has also seen his general practitioner about a generalized rash. His chest X-ray shows multiple soft shadows and a full blood count reveals he has an eosinophilia.

Answers to 9.8

1. **C. Anti-La.** This patient has Sjögren's syndrome, which is associated with many auto-antibodies including some directed against salivary duct epithelium, gastric parietal cells and thyroid tissue. Of the ones listed, anti-La (also termed SS-B) is the most characteristic and occurs in about 50–70% of patients.

2. **B. Anti-Jo-1.** Antibodies to histidyl tRNA synthetase (anti-Jo-1) are associated with myositis, pulmonary fibrosis and Raynaud's phenomenon.

3. **A. Anti-centromere antibodies.** An anti-centromere anti-nucleolar antibody with specificity for a protein of the chromosomal kinetochore is present in the serum of 70% of patients with limited cutaneous systemic sclerosis (CREST syndrome).

4. **I. cANCA.** Some 80% of patients with Wegener's granulomatosis have anti-neutrophil cytoplasmic antibodies. The antibodies against proteinase 3 result in granular staining of the cytoplasm of neutrophils.

5. **J. pANCA.** This patient has polyarteritis nodosa. Antibodies to myeloperoxidase result in perinuclear staining of the cytoplasm of neutrophils.

ABNORMALITIES OF SYNOVIAL FLUID

9.9 **For each of the following descriptions of synovial fluid aspirated from an affected joint, select the most likely diagnosis.**

A   Behçet's disease
B   Gonococcal arthritis
C   Gout
D   Osteoarthrosis
E   Psoriatic arthropathy
F   Pyrophosphate arthropathy
G   Rheumatic fever
H   Rheumatoid arthritis
I   Subacute bacterial endocarditis
J   Septic arthritis

1. The fluid is very turbid and contains >50 000 white cells/mm^2. It has a low viscosity and light microscopy reveals Gram-positive cocci.

2. The fluid is yellow and slightly cloudy with 3000 white cells/mL. Under the polarizing microscope, there are positively birefringent crystals.

3. The fluid is yellow and slightly cloudy with 3000 white cells/mL. Under the polarizing microscope, there are negatively birefringent crystals.

4. The fluid is clear and colourless, with a white cell count of 200/mL. It has a high viscosity.

5. The fluid is very turbid and contains >50 000 white cells/mm^2. It has a low viscosity and light microscopy reveals Gram-negative diplococci.

Answers to 9.9

1. **J. Septic arthritis.** The synovial fluid has many polymorphs and Gram-positive cocci. The organisms commonly responsible for septic arthritis are *Staphylococcus aureus* and *Streptococcus pyogenes.*

2. **F. Pyrophosphate arthropathy.** Pseudogout is due to the deposition of calcium pyrophosphate dihydrate crystals in the synovial space. The crystals are positively birefringent under polarized light.

3. **C. Gout.** Monosodium urate crystals in gout are negatively birefringent.

4. **D. Osteoarthrosis.** The white cell count is slightly elevated but the fluid is of high viscosity.

5. **B. Gonococcal arthritis.** This is the picture of a septic arthritis and the Gram-negative diplococci suggest gonococcal disease.

RHEUMATOLOGICAL DISORDERS

9.10 For each of the following patients, select the most likely rheumatological condition.

A   Chronic discoid lupus
B   CREST syndrome
C   Dermatomyositis
D   Mixed connective tissue disease
E   Morphoea
F   Polymyositis
G   Reiter's syndrome
H   Relapsing polychondritis
I   Systemic lupus erythematosus (SLE)
J   Systemic sclerosis

1.   A 27-year-old African-American complains of alopecia. She has a history of arthritis of the small joints of the hands and depression. She has had two miscarriages.

2.   A 31-year-old Irish woman complains of small joint arthritis, Raynaud's phenomenon, myalgia and muscle weakness. On examination, she has generalized swelling of her fingers. Anti-nuclear factor is positive with very high titres of RNP antibody.

3.   A 40-year-old Welsh man presents with sudden onset of severe pain and swelling in the pinna of the left ear. On examination, he also has nasal tenderness.

4.   A 19-year-old French man presents complaining of dysuria, conjunctivitis and pain in his left knee and right ankle. He has been previously well although he did have to take a few days off work 2 weeks previously with a bout of diarrhoea that settled spontaneously.

5.   A 12-year-old English girl complains of tiredness when climbing stairs. On examination, she has peri-orbital oedema and a violaceous rash on the upper eyelids.

Answers to 9.10

1. **I. Systemic lupus erythematosus (SLE).** This autoimmune disorder is more common in people of African-American descent. Alopecia and small joint arthritis are common presenting features. It is nine times more common in women than in men and the peak age of onset is between 20 and 40 years. The miscarriages are the result of the presence of anti-phospholipid antibodies that predispose to recurrent arterial and venous thrombosis.

2. **D. Mixed connective tissue disease.** This disorder is characterized by the overlap of SLE, systemic sclerosis and myositis. It is associated with high titres of RNP antibodies and often evolves into more classic systemic sclerosis or SLE.

3. **H. Relapsing polychondritis.** This is a disorder characterized by recurrent acute episodes of inflammation and subsequent destruction of cartilage.

4. **G. Reiter's syndrome.** This is the triad of non-specific urethritis, conjunctivitis and reactive arthritis that follows bacterial dysentery or exposure to sexually transmitted infection.

5. **C. Dermatomyositis.** This condition may occur as an isolated syndrome, often in children, or may develop in older patients with an occult neoplasm.

VASCULITIDES

9.11 **For each of the following patients with a vasculitis, select the most likely diagnosis.**

A   Churg–Strauss syndrome
B   Cutaneous leucocytoclastic angiitis
C   Essential mixed cryoglobulinaemia
D   Henoch–Schönlein purpura
E   Kawasaki disease
F   Polyarteritis nodosa
G   Systemic sclerosis
H   Takayasu's arteritis
I   Temporal arteritis
J   Wegener's granulomatosis

1.   A 52-year-old man presents with itching, palpable purpura and urticaria. The symptoms respond to antihistamines. Auto-antibody tests show he is ANCA positive at high titre.

2.   An 8-year-old boy complains of abdominal pain and pain in both knees after an apparently trivial upper respiratory tract infection. Two days later, he develops a purpuric rash on both his legs.

3.   A 4-year-old boy presents with a 1-week history of fever, conjunctival infection, red lips, mouth and tongue and desquamation of the palms and soles.

4.   A 49-year-old man presents with abdominal pain, palpable urticaria and shortness of breath. His blood pressure is 210/140 mmHg. His medical history includes ischaemic heart disease and hepatitis B.

5.   A 38-year-old woman presents with painful joints and purpura. On examination, she has cervical, axillary and inguinal lymphadenopathy. Her medical history includes hepatitis C infection.

Answers to 9.11

1. **B. Cutaneous leucocytoclastic angiitis.** Urticaria and palpable purpura that respond to antihistamines are typical of this rare disorder.

2. **D. Henoch–Schönlein purpura.** This is also referred to as anaphylactoid purpura and in most cases is a self-limiting condition that may follow respiratory tract infections in childhood. It may also occur in adults. It is a distinct systemic vasculitic syndrome and is characterized by palpable purpura (mostly occurring on the buttocks and legs), arthralgias, gastrointestinal symptoms and glomerulonephritis.

3. **E. Kawasaki disease.** Although it may resemble self-limiting viral infections of childhood (which can also lead to skin desquamation), this is an important diagnosis not to miss since the associated coronary artery aneurysms (in about 25% of cases) may be fatal if the condition is left untreated. Apart from this complication, the prognosis is excellent. High-dose intravenous gammaglobulin together with aspirin have been shown to be effective in reducing the coronary artery abnormalities.

4. **F. Polyarteritis nodosa.** There is an association with previous hepatitis B infection. It is a multisystem, necrotizing vasculitis of small- and medium-sized arteries involving the kidneys and other viscera. The presentation is usually with vague and non-specific symptoms. During the course of the illness, the patient may develop arthralgia, hypertension, renal failure, peripheral neuropathy, abdominal pain, purpura, cutaneous infarcts, congestive cardiac failure and strokes.

5. **C. Essential mixed cryoglobulinaemia.** This presents with arthralgia and purpura. There is a strong association with hepatitis C infection. The condition may present as a predominantly cutaneous vasculitis but it can be associated with glomerulonephritis, arthralgia, hepatosplenomegaly and lymphadenopathy.

BONE DISEASE

9.12 For each of the following patients, select the most likely bone disease.

A   Acropachy
B   Hypertrophic pulmonary osteoarthropathy
C   Osteoarthritis
D   Osteomalacia
E   Osteopetrosis
F   Osteoporosis
G   Paget's disease
H   Pathological fracture
I   Psoriatic arthropathy
J   Rickets

1.   A 70-year-old woman complains of difficulty in climbing stairs and of pain in her hips, knees and shoulder girdles. Radiological investigation reveals Looser's zones in the pubic rami.

2.   A 54-year-old man complains of sudden-onset pain in his thoracic spine. On examination, he looks thin and unwell. There is tenderness on palpation of the 8th thoracic vertebral body.

3.   A 50-year-old man complains of pain in both wrists and forearms. On examination, there is finger clubbing and the forearms are very tender on palpation.

4.   An 82-year-old woman attempts to stand after sitting in a chair, hears a clicking sound and falls to the floor.

5.   A 30-year-old woman is admitted to hospital with a Bell's palsy. The skull X-ray shows marked thickening of the skull vault.

Answers to 9.12

1. **D. Osteomalacia.** Multiple aches and pains are characteristic of this condition as is the proximal muscle weakness that causes difficulty in climbing stairs. Looser's zones, 'pseudofractures', or Milkman's fractures are focal radiolucent bands that may be found along the concave side of the femoral neck, the pubic rami, the ribs, the clavicles and the scapulae. They are a feature of advanced osteomalacia (and rickets) and may be absent in less severe cases.

2. **H. Pathological fracture.** The pain is of sudden onset suggesting an acute cause. Tenderness on palpation of T8 raises the possibility of collapse/fracture and in a thin, unwell-looking patient, a pathological fracture (e.g. due to metastatic disease) should be considered.

3. **B. Hypertrophic pulmonary osteoarthropathy (HPOA).** Patients with a wide range of pulmonary, hepatic and intestinal disorders may develop digital clubbing. In some cases, this is associated with HPOA where there is marked tenderness of the lower ends of the radius and ulnar. X-rays show subperiosteal new bone formation. Bronchogenic carcinoma (except the small cell variety) is the most common cause of HPOA with clubbing. The other causes of HPOA include pleural tumours, lung abscesses and empyemas. HPOA may occur without finger clubbing in chronic liver disease and occasionally in inflammatory bowel disease.

4. **F. Osteoporosis.** Elderly patients with severe osteoporosis may suffer a fractured neck of femur with minimal trauma; in some cases, the fracture occurs simply on trying to stand. The fracture is, in one sense, a pathological fracture in that it occurs through abnormal bone but since osteoporosis would seem to be the direct cause in this patient, it is considered to be the best answer.

5. **E. Osteopetrosis.** Several types of osteopetrosis (Albers–Schönberg disease, marble bone disease) are known to exist. There is defective resorption of bone by osteoclasts leading to thickened bones. In the severe, autosomal recessive form (osteopetrosis congenital) the marrow space is replaced with bone, which results in anaemia, infection and early death. In the less severe, autosomal dominant variety (osteopetrosis tarda) the condition is usually detected in family studies or as an incidental radiological finding. In the skull, the thickened bone may lead to compression neuropathies. The molecular defects of some cases have recently been identified (e.g. deficiency in cathepsin K).

COMPLICATIONS OF FRACTURES

9.13 **For each of the following patients who have had a bone fracture, select the most likely complication.**

A Compartment syndrome
B Deep vein thrombosis
C Fat embolism
D Growth arrest
E Hypovolaemic shock
F Malunion
G Non-union
H Osteoarthritis
I Osteomyelitis
J Post-traumatic reflex dystrophy

1. A 21-year-old man is a front-seat passenger involved in a road traffic accident. When he arrives at the hospital, he has a compound fracture of the left humerus and both lower limbs are extended and rotated. He is unconscious with a pulse of 130 bpm and a blood pressure of 70/50 mmHg.

2. A 34-year-old builder is injured at work after his right arm is trapped by a piece of machinery. He is taken to hospital but discharges himself. The following day he returns with severe pain in his forearm. On examination, the anterior aspect of the forearm is bruised, swollen and tender and he is unable to flex his wrist.

3. A 27-year-old woman has a fall while skiing and sustains a compound fracture of the left tibia. It is internally fixed and, after several weeks, she seems to be recovering well. However, some months later she has a persistent discharge from a sinus on the left leg. Oral antibiotics seem to settle the problem but it recurs as soon as they are stopped.

4. A 7-year-old boy falls down a well and suffers a fracture of his right femoral epiphysis. The following year, his parents are concerned that he has a persistent limp on walking.

5. A 40-year-old man trips in the street and fractures his right ankle. The following week, he complains of increasing swelling in the right leg. On examination, the left leg and thigh are swollen and the limb feels warm with dilated superficial veins.

Answers to 9.13

1. **E. Hypovolaemic shock.** The patient has a tachycardia and is hypotensive after trauma and blood loss must be the first consideration. The lower limbs are extended and rotated, suggesting fractures involving the femur or acetabulum. These may result in considerable 'internal' bleeding.

2. **A. Compartment syndrome.** The muscles of the forearm are contained in a fibrous fascial compartment. Swelling of the muscle due to ischaemia or bleeding within the compartment causes a vicious circle of compression and further ischaemia. If the pressure is not relieved (e.g. by a fasciotomy), the muscles will die and fibrose, leading to permanent deformity and weakness of the hand (Volkmann's ischaemic contracture).

3. **I. Osteomyelitis.** Infection within the bone is extremely difficult to eradicate. The discharging sinus may heal over but breaks down again or new ones develop because of the persisting source of infection in the bone. Prolonged courses of fusidic acid may help to resolve the condition but surgical removal of the infected bone may be required.

4. **D. Growth arrest.** A fracture through an epiphysis is uncommon in childhood but may result in the premature arrest of bone growth. The limp on walking is due to the unequal lower limb lengths.

5. **B. Deep vein thrombosis.** Deep vein thrombosis is a common complication of immobility following a lower limb fracture and requires urgent treatment to reduce the risk of post-thrombotic syndrome and pulmonary embolus. Diagnosis on clinical grounds alone is difficult but a warm, swollen limb with dilated superficial veins merits anticoagulation with heparin pending confirmation of the diagnosis with Doppler ultrasound or a venogram.

Nervous system

LOCATION OF NEUROLOGICAL LESIONS

10.1 Select the most likely site of the neurological lesion in each of the following patients with a neurological deficit.

A Left cerebellar hemisphere
B Left frontal lobe
C Left parietal lobe
D Left temporal lobe
E Mid-brain
F Occipital lobe
G Right cerebellar hemisphere
H Right frontal lobe
I Right parietal lobe
J Right temporal lobe

1. A right-handed patient presents with a global dysphasia.

2. A right-handed patient presents with dressing apraxia.

3. A right-handed patient presents with visual agnosia.

4. A left-handed patient presents with rigidity and bradykinesia.

5. A right-handed patient presents with intention tremor and past pointing affecting his right upper limb and impaired heel–shin testing in his right lower limb.

Answers to 10.1

1. **C. Left parietal lobe.** The language centres are situated in the dominant cerebral hemisphere.

2. **I. Right parietal lobe.** Spatial awareness and organization are situated in the non-dominant hemisphere.

3. **F. Occipital lobe.** This area controls visual processing.

4. **E. Mid-brain.** The patient has extra-pyramidal signs as, for example, in Parkinson's disease, where the defect is in the substantia nigra of the mid-brain.

5. **G. Right cerebellar hemisphere.** The patient has right-sided cerebellar signs and the ipsilateral cerebellar hemisphere is therefore at fault.

THE GLASGOW COMA SCALE

10.2 **For each of the following scenarios, select the correct Glasgow Coma Scale score.**

A   3
B   4
C   5
D   6
E   7
F   9
G   10
H   11
I   13
J   14

1.   A patient who had no eye opening, no verbal responses and extends to pain.

2.   A patient who responds to pain by opening the eyes, has confused speech but localizes the painful stimulus.

3.   A patient who opens the eyes to command, but whose best verbal response is the use of inappropriate words and withdraws the limbs from painful stimuli.

4.   A patient who spontaneously opens the eyes, obeys commands by appropriate motor responses but whose conversation is confused.

5.   A patient who opens the eyes to painful stimuli but responds with abnormal limb flexion and makes incomprehensible sounds.

Answers to 10.2

The Glasgow Coma Scale scores eye opening, verbal responses and best motor responses. The minimum score is 3 and the maximum 15.

Eye opening: none = 1, to pain = 2, to speech = 3, spontaneously = 4

Verbal response: none = 1, incomprehensible sounds = 2, inappropriate words = 3, confused conversation = 4, orientated = 5

Best motor responses: none = 1, extension = 2, abnormal flexion = 3, withdrawal = 4, localizes stimulus = 5, obeys commands = 6

1. **B.** Glasgow Coma Scale of 4.

2. **H.** Glasgow Coma Scale of 11.

3. **G.** Glasgow Coma Scale of 10.

4. **J.** Glasgow Coma Scale of 14.

5. **E.** Glasgow Coma Scale of 7.

MOVEMENT DISORDERS

10.3 **For each of the scenarios outlined below, select the most appropriate diagnosis of the movement disorder.**

A   Cerebellar tremor
B   Essential tremor
C   Hemidystonia
D   Hemifacial spasm
E   Huntington's disease
F   Segmental dystocia
G   Sydenham's chorea
H   Tardive dyskinesia
I   Tic
J   Wilson's disease

1. A 69-year-old woman with a long history of chronic schizophrenia is noted to have continuous involuntary movements of the orobuccolingual and masticatory muscles.

2. A 40-year-old man is referred to hospital with a history of recurrent falls. He used to work in an office but was sacked because of his poor work earlier in the year and he admits to increasing forgetfulness. On examination, he has brief, shock-like movements of his limbs. His brother suffers from similar symptoms but they are both adopted so no other family history is available.

3. A 59-year-old woman complains of shaking in her arms and difficulty in walking. She has had to stop sewing as she finds it impossible to thread the needle. There is no tremor at rest. On finger-nose testing, she starts confidently but the nearer she gets to the target, the more obvious the tremor becomes.

4. A 53-year-old man attends the surgery with his wife who is concerned that he is always moving his head and cannot keep still. On examination, he has repetitive, rapid, brief jerks of his head that occur every few minutes. When they are brought to his attention, he can concentrate hard and suppress them for a short while but then he feels them start again.

5. A 47-year-old woman is admitted to hospital after falling in the street. She says one of her legs just gave way under her. Her husband complains that she thrashes around in bed, sometimes kicking him violently. As she is being observed, her right arm and leg suddenly jerk out violently without warning.

Answers to 10.3

1. **H. Tardive dyskinesia.** As many as 20% of patients taking long-term antipsychotics develop a syndrome of involuntary movements centred around the mouth, lips and tongue.

2. **E. Huntington's disease.** This is an autosomal dominant disorder due to the inheritance of an expanded triplicate repeat. Onset is typically in the 30s or 40s with chorea, tics or myoclonus associated with psychiatric disturbance and dementia.

3. **A. Cerebellar tremor.** Cerebellar lesions cause tremor on movement rather than at rest (intention tremor, past pointing, dysdiadokinesis). The associated ataxia may make walking difficult and lead to falls.

4. **I. Tic.** A tic is an involuntary movement that the person can suppress with conscious effort for a short period of time. Trying to suppress the movement can cause distress that is immediately relieved once the motion occurs.

5. **C. Hemidystonia or hemiballismus.** This may be due to a lesion in the contralateral thalamus.

CAUSES OF ATAXIA

10.4 **For each of the patients described below, select the most likely cause of their ataxia from the list given.**

A   Adverse drug reaction
B   Alcohol
C   Friedreich's ataxia
D   Miller–Fisher syndrome
E   Multiple sclerosis
F   Paraneoplastic syndrome
G   Pernicious anaemia
H   Prion disease
I   Syphilis
J   Von Hippel–Lindau disease

1. A 20-year-old woman is admitted to hospital in a confused state. Her partner says that she has been complaining of headache and vomiting for 12 h and was unsteady on her feet before the collapse. He knows she had some sort of treatment to her eyes when she was younger. On examination, fundoscopy reveals multiple vascular abnormalities and laser burns.

2. An 18-year-old boy is referred to hospital because he has been progressively more clumsy on walking for 2–3 years. On examination, he is ataxic, has absent ankle jerks but bilaterally extensor plantar reflexes.

3. A 21-year-old man is admitted to hospital complaining of unsteadiness and double vision that came on rapidly a few hours previously. He has just finished a short course of ciprofloxacin for a diarrhoeal illness. He admits to drinking 10–12 pints of beer several times a week. On examination, he is ataxic, has impaired eye movements and all the limb reflexes are either absent or very weak.

4. A 27-year-old woman presents with a 2-day history of unsteadiness and difficulty with fine movements such as writing. Several years previously, she had a similar episode associated with diplopia that almost completely resolved over several weeks. She says she only drinks alcohol at weekends and is on no medication apart from the oral contraceptive pill. On examination, she is ataxic, has a left-sided intention tremor and dysdiadokinesis.

5. A 66-year-old man complains of increasing unsteadiness over the last 3 months. He has a history of bipolar affective disorder for which he takes fluoxetine. He is an ex-smoker with a chronic cough and drinks 20 units of alcohol a week. Investigations include a normal B_{12} and folate level, a negative VDRL but strongly positive anti-Hu antibodies in his CSF.

Answers to 10.4

1. **J. Von Hippel–Lindau disease.** This is an autosomal dominant disorder due to mutations in the VHL gene on chromosome 3. Characteristic features include cerebellar and retinal haemangioblastomas, renal and pancreatic cysts and an increased risk of renal cell carcinoma. This patient had her retinal haemangioblastomas treated by photocoagulation but subsequently bled from a small cerebellar lesion.

2. **C. Friedreich's ataxia.** This is an autosomal dominant disorder due to a trinucleotide repeat expansion in the frataxin gene. It is associated with progressive loss of the dorsal sensory columns in the spinal cord, and subsequent loss of joint position sense. Other features include optic atrophy, diabetes and cardiomyopathy.

3. **D. Miller–Fisher syndrome.** This disorder, a variant of Guillain–Barré syndrome, presents with acute ataxia, ophthalmoplegia and areflexia following a diarrhoeal illness. If a lumbar puncture is performed, the CSF fluid pressure may be raised and the fluid contains antibodies against a membrane-bound protein of the myelin sheath. Ciprofloxacin is not a commonly recognized cause of ataxia.

4. **E. Multiple sclerosis.** The acute relapsing history and lesions occurring in more than one component of the central nervous system are typical of this disorder.

5. **F. Paraneoplastic syndrome.** This man had a small cell lung cancer. Sometimes the chest X-ray appears normal and the underlying diagnosis is not obvious. However, anti-Hu antibodies in the CSF in this case point to the correct diagnosis.

MUSCULAR DYSTROPHIES

10.5 **Below is a list of muscle disorders. For each of the following scenarios, select the correct diagnosis.**

A   Becker's muscular dystrophy
B   Central core disease
C   Charcot–Marie–Tooth disease
D   Duchenne's muscular dystrophy
E   Emery–Dreifuss muscular dystrophy
F   Fascio-scapulohumeral dystrophy
G   Limb girdle dystrophy
H   McArdle's disease
I   Myoclonus, epilepsy and ragged red fibres
J   Myotonic dystrophy

1.   A teenager complains of severe pain and cramp in both his legs whenever he is made to do sport at school. The symptoms are so severe he often has to stop running and walk slowly. He has noticed that, if he does carry on exercising, the symptoms do improve and he is then able to run with less discomfort.

2.   A 39-year-old man is seen in the ophthalmology clinic before cataract surgery. He denies any specific symptoms apart from gradual visual loss. However, on examination, his face looks rather drawn, he has bilateral ptosis and frontal balding.

3.   A 5-year-old boy presents with delay in achieving his motor milestones. He complains of pain in his legs when walking in school. Over the next 2 years, he develops progressive muscle weakness, eventually finding it difficult to climb stairs and then even to stand up.

4.   A 47-year-old man develops progressive muscle weakness in the upper and lower limbs. When asked to grip an object tightly, he finds it difficult to let go quickly. He says that his mother suffered from a mitochondrial disorder.

5.   A 25-year-old woman develops progressive muscle weakness, first in the face and then spreading to the shoulders but with sparing of the extraocular, pharyngeal and lingual muscles. When asked to stand up, face a wall and push hard against it with her hands, the scapulae rise up, almost over her shoulders. She recalls her father suffered from mitochondrial encephalomyopathy.

Answers to 10.5

1. **H. McArdle's disease.** This is an autosomal recessive disorder due to mutations in myophosphorylase (on chromosome 11q). The muscles cannot use stored glycogen for energy during vigorous exercise. If exercise continues, alternative sources of energy are used by muscle so the symptoms tend to abate.

2. **J. Myotonic dystrophy.** This is an autosomal dominant disorder characterized by the features listed and also diabetes, hypogonadism and sometimes mental retardation. A characteristic myotonic feature of the condition is that the patient can grip strongly but is unable to relax the grip quickly. It is due to inheritance of an expanded trinucleotide repeat sequence on chromosome 19q.

3. **D. Duchenne's muscular dystrophy.** This is an X-linked recessive disorder that presents in early childhood with progressive muscle weakness. Fibrosis and fat infiltration produce characteristically enlarged gastrocnemius muscles. Respiratory muscle weakness and death usually occur in early adult life.

4. **I. Myoclonus, epilepsy and ragged red fibres.** This is a mitochondrial DNA defect and therefore maternally inherited. The ragged red fibres on muscle biopsy represent myocytes with large numbers of abnormal mitochondria. Other mitochondrial disorders include Kearns Sayre syndrome, Leber's hereditary optic neuropathy and MELAS (mitochondrial encephalomyopathy, lactic acidosis and stroke-like episodes).

5. **F. Fascio-scapulohumeral dystrophy.** This is an autosomal dominant disorder that usually presents in early adult life with progressive muscle weakness. Winging of the scapulae occurs because of weakness of serratus anterior muscles. The history of mitochondrial disease in the father is irrelevant since these disorders can only be transmitted by affected mothers.

MEMORY LOSS

10.6 **For each of the following presentations, select the most likely cause.**

A   Alzheimer's disease
B   Cerebral metastases
C   Chronic subdural haematoma
D   Depression
E   Expressive dysphasia
F   Hypothyroidism
G   Lewy Body dementia
H   Muti-infarct dementia
I   Normal pressure hydrocephalus
J   Wernicke–Korsakoff syndrome

1.   A 45-year-old woman is brought in by her husband complaining that she forgets things and then insists that she does not. When asked what she had for breakfast she gave a credible list of juice, cereal, toast, bacon, egg and tea, but according to her husband, she had only had a cup of tea and toast. There is a history of alcohol abuse but she adamantly denies it. Examination reveals memory impairment, nystagmus, diplopia, ataxia and peripheral neuropathy.

2.   A 55-year-old man is admitted to hospital with a 6-month history of incontinence and increasing unsteadiness on his feet. Apart from an apraxic gait and Mini-Mental State Examination (MMSE) score of 15/30, no abnormality is found.

3.   An 80-year-old woman is brought to her general practitioner by her husband who is concerned because she wanders out of her home and then loses her way. He has noticed a gradual deterioration in her memory over the last 3 years. She is able to talk about her childhood but is unable to recall any recent events.

4.   A 70-year-old woman presents with weight gain, constipation and lethargy. Initial tests show haemoglobin of 13 g/dL, MCV of 106 fL and MMSE of 20/30.

5.   An 82-year-old man with ischaemic heart disease and hypertension is admitted to hospital with a 12-month history of increasing forgetfulness and confusion for the last 3 days, which followed a 'funny turn' while eating his dinner. His wife says that he had two episodes of confusion associated with a disturbance of speech during the last year.

Answers to 10.6

1. **J. Wernicke–Korsakoff syndrome.** This patient has a typical triad of ocular signs, ataxia and impaired memory. Some patients with this syndrome confabulate and insert false but credible information to fill in their memory gaps. It is caused by thiamine deficiency affecting the midline limbic structures that results from heavy dependence on alcohol and the concomitant poor diet. This patient's peripheral neuropathy is also due to alcohol abuse.

2. **I. Normal pressure hydrocephalus.** The diagnosis is easily made in the presence of the well-known triad of dementia, unsteady gait and urinary incontinence. In contrast to Alzheimer's disease, the last two symptoms occur early in normal pressure hydrocephalus. The CSF pressure and composition are normal.

3. **A. Alzheimer's disease.** A gradual and global deterioration of this patient's cognitive function with advancing age suggests the diagnosis. The patients are unable to learn and retain recent information and there is a gradual deterioration of language and motor functions. Behaviour changes are common and include wandering, aggression, agitation and paranoia.

4. **F. Hypothyroidism.** The clinical features of this patient suggest a diagnosis of hypothyroidism with probable co-existent pernicious anaemia, although a raised MCV may be found in patients without obvious B_{12} deficiency on laboratory testing. A variety of central nervous system disorders have been described in this condition, including dementia, epilepsy, drop attacks, cerebellar ataxia and peripheral neuropathy.

5. **H. Multi-infarct (vascular) dementia.** Vascular dementia culminates after a single major stroke or following a succession of transient ischaemic attacks, manifesting as brief episodes of loss of consciousness, impairment of memory, visual loss or motor dysfunction. Vascular dementia results from involvement of several vessels supplying the cerebral cortex and subcortical structures.

NEUROLOGICAL DEFICITS

10.7 **For each of the following patients with a neurological deficit, select the most appropriate description.**

A   Cerebellar lesion
B   Extrapyramidal lesion
C   Gait apraxia
D   Hypertrophic neuropathy
E   Marche á petits pas
F   Mononeuritis multiplex
G   Mononeuropathy
H   Proximal myopathy
I   Sensory ataxia
J   Upper motor neurone lesion

1.   A patient with Bell's palsy but no other neurological signs.

2.   An elderly patient walks with a broad-based gait, taking short steps and placing his feet flat on the ground like a person walking on ice. He cannot hop on one foot but neurological examination does not reveal any consistent motor or sensory deficits.

3.   A patient who complains of difficulty in climbing stairs and in standing from a crouched position.

4.   A patient with a positive Romberg's sign.

5.   A patient with tremor, bradykinesia and cog-wheel rigidity.

Answers to 10.7

1. **G. Mononeuropathy.** The VIIth cranial nerve is affected.

2. **C. Gait apraxia.** This is also called 'magnetic gait'. The patient usually has frontal lobe signs including dementia and grasp and suck reflexes. The most common cause is a degenerative process such as Alzheimer's disease. Other causes include subdural haematoma, tumours and normal-pressure hydrocephalus.

3. **H. Proximal myopathy.** The pelvic girdle muscles and quadriceps are required for climbing stairs and standing from a crouched position. The causes include osteomalacia, Cushing's syndrome, carcinomatous myopathy and Graves' disease.

4. **I. Sensory ataxia.** Romberg's sign is positive when a patient is more unsteady with their eyes shut than with them open whilst standing upright. By shutting the eyes, the patient loses visual clues that help to maintain balance. Sensory examination will reveal loss of joint position and vibration sense.

5. **B. Extrapyramidal lesion.** The extrapyramidal system helps to integrate motor activity. These are the typical signs of Parkinson's disease.

SLEEP DISTURBANCE

10.8 Select the most appropriate description of the sleep disturbance described in the following scenarios.

A   Cataplexy
B   Day-time somnolence
C   Hypnagogic hallucinations
D   Night terrors
E   Nocturnal fits
F   Sleep attacks
G   Sleep paralysis
H   Sleep talking
I   Sleep walking
J   Transient global amnesia

1.   A patient who is about to fall asleep is noted to suddenly startle and jerk himself awake.

2.   A patient who is told some bad news suddenly falls to the ground asleep.

3.   A patient who is asleep is noticed to be jerking all four limbs but is unrousable.

4.   A patient who wakes screaming after being noted to be asleep.

5.   A patient who recounts being unable to move after waking in the middle of the night.

Answers to 10.8

1. **C. Hypnagogic hallucinations.** These are brief episodes during the transition between wakefulness and sleep. The hallucinations are vivid perceptions (auditory or visual) that appear particularly while drifting into sleep. These may occur in normal people, especially if sleep deprived.

2. **A. Cataplexy.** This is the sudden loss of muscle tone precipitated by strong emotion, surprise or even laughter. The severity of the attacks ranges from light knee buckling or drooping of the jaw to complete collapse. Some benefit with clomipramine has been reported.

3. **E. Nocturnal fits.** However deeply asleep, people are normally rousable, even if it takes some effort. If a patient is unrousable it suggests the person is comatose or having a fit.

4. **D. Night terrors.** These are more common in children but some drugs may precipitate attacks in adults, e.g. L-DOPA. There is usually a family history of sleep walking or night terrors.

5. **G. Sleep paralysis.** This consists of a transient experience during which the patient is unable to move any muscle but breathes normally. These attacks may occur in normal people. Sometimes it is difficult to decide whether people were really awake during their period of paralysis or whether they dreamt they had been awake and unable to move.

NERVE INJURIES

10.9 **For each of the following patients, who have sustained a neurological lesion, select the most likely diagnosis.**

A   Common peroneal nerve lesion
B   Damage to lower trunk of brachial plexus
C   Damage to upper trunk of brachial plexus
D   Dupuytren's contracture
E   Femoral nerve lesion
F   Median nerve lesion
G   Meralgia paraesthetica
H   Radial nerve lesion
I   T1 lesion
J   Ulnar nerve lesion

1.   A 19-year-old man complains of tingling and numbness on the inner side of his right forearm and right little, ring and middle fingers. On examination, the small muscles of the right hand appear wasted.

2.   A 23-year-old woman suffers a fracture of the humerus while skiing. She subsequently seeks medical attention because she cannot use her hand properly.

3.   A 46-year-old policeman attends his general practitioner because he has developed pain and tingling in his right thigh. The symptoms are worse on standing and relieved by sitting down. On examination, there is diminished light touch sensation over the anterolateral aspect of the thigh.

4.   The mother of a 3-month-old baby is concerned because she has noticed that one of his arms 'looks twisted' and seems to hang lower than the other and the baby does not bend the elbow.

5.   A 60-year-old housewife is noted to have a 'claw hand'. On examination, there is a flexion deformity at the metacarpophalangeal and proximal interphalangeal joints of the middle, ring and little fingers. The distal interphalangeal joints are spared and there is no sensory loss.

Answers to 10.9

1.   **I. T1 lesion.** The patient has sensory loss in the distribution of the T1 dermatome and T1 innervates all the small muscles of the hand. Possible causes include a cervical rib, neurofibroma, syringomyelia, cervical spondylosis or previous shoulder dislocation.

2.   **H. Radial nerve lesion.** The radial nerve may be damaged by a fracture of the humerus involving the spiral groove. The hand cannot be used properly because of wrist drop.

3.   **G. Meralgia paraesthetica.** This is due to compression of the lateral cutaneous nerve of the thigh, often as it emerges beneath the inguinal ligament. It may occur in obese, pregnant women and athletes and also those wearing tight or heavy belts (such as this policeman).

4.   **C. Damage to upper trunk of brachial plexus.** This is Erb's paralysis. There is damage to C5 and C6 and paralysis of biceps (inability to flex elbow), supinator (forearm pronated), deltoid (arm hangs vertically), brachialis, brachioradialis, supraspinatus and infraspinatus (arm internally rotated).

5.   **D. Dupuytren's contracture.** The differential diagnosis of a 'claw hand' also includes ulnar nerve lesions. The lack of sensory loss and sparing of the distal interphalangeal joints makes Dupuytren's contracture the correct diagnosis in this case.

EPONYMOUS NEUROLOGICAL SYNDROMES

10.10 For each of the following constellations of neurological deficits, select the correct eponymous neurological syndrome.

A   Brown–Sequard
B   Claude
C   Collet–Sicard
D   Eaton–Lambert
E   Guillain–Barré
F   Millard–Gubler
G   Parinaud
H   Villaret
I   Wallenberg
J   Weber

1. An ipsilateral IIIrd nerve palsy with contralateral cerebellar signs.

2. Ipsilateral Vth, IXth, Xth and XIth nerve palsies and ipsilateral Horner's and cerebellar signs with contralateral spinothalamic tract signs.

3. Ipsilateral VIth and lower motor neurone VIIth nerve palsies and a contralateral hemiplegia.

4. Ipsilateral IXth, Xth, XIth and XIIth lower motor neurone palsies.

5. An ipsilateral IIIrd nerve palsy with contralateral upper motor neurone facial palsy and contralateral hemiplegia.

Answers to 10.10

1.   **B. Claude.** The lesion is in the cerebral peduncle and involves the red nucleus.

2.   **I. Wallenberg.** The lesion is in the lateral medulla, hence the other name for this condition, lateral medullary syndrome.

3.   **F. Millard–Gubler.** The lesion is in the pontomedullary junction.

4.   **C. Collet–Sicard.** The lesion is just outside the skull at the jugular foramen and is likely to involve the XIIth nerve as well as the three nerves (IXth, Xth and XIth) that lie in the jugular foramen.

5.   **J. Weber.** The lesion is in the anterior cerebral peduncle.

NEUROSURGERY

10.11 **For each of the following patients with a neurosurgical disorder, select the most likely diagnosis.**

A   Acute subdural haemorrhage
B   Cerebral abscess
C   Chronic subdural haemorrhage
D   Communicating hydrocephalus
E   Extradural haemorrhage
F   Meningioma
G   Non-communicating hydrocephalus
H   Pituitary apoplexy
I   Schwannoma
J   Subarachnoid haemorrhage

1. A 70-year-old man presents to his general practitioner complaining of episodes of dizziness. On examination, he has nystagmus of gaze to the left and right and an absent right corneal reflex. An X-ray of the skull shows expansion of the internal auditory meatus.

2. A 56-year-old woman is admitted to hospital with sudden onset of severe headache. On examination, her pulse is 120 bpm and her blood pressure is 90/60 mmHg. She is too unwell to give a full history but says that she had some flashing lights in her eyes just before the headache started and that now she cannot see at all.

3. The police take a 19-year-old man to hospital after he is found on the street. It appears that he may have been the victim of an assault but he is intoxicated and will not cooperate with a physical examination. His condition rapidly deteriorates and an urgent CT scan is performed. This is reported as showing blood in the basal cisterns and a small contusion in the left frontal lobe. A lumbar puncture reveals >1000 red cells and xanthochromia.

4. A 64-year-old woman presents following a seizure. She has never had fits before but does recall being admitted for observation after a road traffic accident several years previously. On examination, there are no abnormal physical signs. A CT scan shows a 6×4 cm midline lesion arising in the superior sagittal sinus and compressing the frontal lobes.

5. An 18-year-old man with spina bifida is admitted to hospital complaining of increasing headaches. His parents say that as a child he had a ventriculoperitoneal shunt inserted to relieve pressure around his brain. On examination, he has bilateral papilloedema.

Answers to 10.11

1.   **I. Schwannoma.** This is also termed an acoustic neuroma and is occasionally associated with phaeochromocytomas. The tumour grows in the cerebellar-pontine angle and may result in Vth, VIIth and VIIIth cranial nerve lesions. Loss of the corneal reflex is an early clinical sign. The nystagmus is not usually sustained and may be either cerebellar or vestibular in origin.

2.   **H. Pituitary apoplexy.** The history given could be of a subarachnoid haemorrhage; however, the sudden bilateral visual loss suggests a lesion in close proximity to the optic tracts.

3.   **J. Subarachnoid haemorrhage.** This unfortunate man suffered a subarachnoid haemorrhage while out drinking, collapsed and hit his head. Although the initial history suggests an acute extradural or subdural, the diagnosis is made clear by the CT scan and lumbar puncture.

4.   **F. Meningioma.** These tumours are more common in females than males. Other common sites include the olfactory groove, base of the skull, lateral ventricles and within the spinal canal. *Note* that, as in this patient, the absence of papilloedema does not exclude significant raised intracranial pressure.

5.   **G. Non-communicating hydrocephalus.** Spina bifida is frequently associated with the Arnold–Chiari malformation, where there is congenital downward protrusion of the cerebellum into the foramen magnum and occlusion of the foramina of the fourth ventricle. The CSF cannot escape into the basal cisterns. The condition is often treated with a shunt in childhood but these shunts may block, causing a raised intracranial pressure in later life.

Haematology

HAEMATOLOGICAL INVESTIGATIONS

11.1 For each of the following patients, select the most likely finding from the analysis of the peripheral blood.

A   Anaemia
B   Lymphocytosis
C   Lymphopenia
D   Neutropenia
E   Neutrophilia
F   Pancytopenia
G   Polycythaemia
H   Reticulocytosis
I   Thrombocytopenia
J   Thrombocytosis

1.   A patient with infectious mononucleosis.

2.   A patient who has just started treatment with B_{12} and folate for megaloblastic anaemia.

3.   A patient with chronic renal failure.

4.   A patient with chronic obstructive pulmonary disease.

5.   A patient with disseminated intravascular coagulation.

Answers to 11.1

1. **B. Lymphocytosis.** Many viral infections, including infectious mononucleosis, cause a lymphocytosis.

2. **H. Reticulocytosis.** The administration of haematinics results in a brisk increase in erythropoiesis with a transient rise in the peripheral blood reticulocyte count.

3. **A. Anaemia.** There are several mechanisms that may result in anaemia in patients with chronic renal failure, the most important being a reduced production of erythropoietin. Other mechanisms include iron deficiency due to blood loss from the gastrointestinal or genitourinary tracts, folate loss into the dialysate and shortened red cell survival.

4. **G. Polycythaemia.** Chronic hypoxia stimulates the production of erythropoietin causing an increase in the red cell mass.

5. **I. Thrombocytopenia.** The intravascular coagulation depletes peripheral blood of platelets.

ANAEMIA

11.2 **For each of the following patients, select the most likely cause of their anaemia.**

A   Aplastic anaemia
B   Folic acid deficiency
C   Iron deficiency
D   Multiple myelomatosis
E   Myelofibrosis
F   Peptic ulcer disease
G   Pernicious anaemia
H   Rheumatoid arthritis
I   Vitamin B_{12} deficiency
J   Vitamin C deficiency

1.   A 60-year-old woman with a history of thyrotoxicosis complains of easy bruising and recurrent blood blisters in her mouth. Her white cell count is 2×10^9/L, platelets 20×10^9/L and the haemoglobin is 6 g/dL.

2.   A 35-year-old woman with irregular periods complains of fatigue. Investigations show that she has a haemoglobin of 8 g/dL with a low mean corpuscular volume and a low mean corpuscular haemoglobin concentration. Gastroscopy is normal.

3.   A 65-year-old man complains of low back pain and fatigue. He has a haemoglobin of 9 g/dL with a normal mean corpuscular volume and mean corpuscular haemoglobin concentration. His ESR is 120 mm/h.

4.   A 70-year-old woman has stiffness, pain and swelling of her wrists and knees. She also complains of fatigue and easy bruising. She has a haemoglobin of 9 g/dL with a normal mean corpuscular volume and mean corpuscular haemoglobin concentration. Her ESR is 80 mm/h.

5.   A 38-year-old woman who had a resection of her terminal ileum for Crohn's disease 6 years ago presents with breathlessness and fatigue. She has a megaloblastic anaemia with a haemoglobin concentration of 7 g/dL.

Answers to 11.2

1. **A. Aplastic anaemia.** This patient's pancytopenia suggests marrow failure (aplastic anaemia). A haemorrhagic tendency is the most common presentation of this disorder. In about half the cases, a history of exposure to an incriminating agent may be forthcoming. The history of thyrotoxicosis was relevant in that this woman was taking carbimazole.

2. **C. Iron deficiency.** This patient's irregular periods are probably caused by menorrhagia resulting in excessive blood loss and iron deficiency anaemia. The low mean corpuscular volume and mean corpuscular haemoglobin concentration are in keeping with that diagnosis.

3. **D. Multiple myelomatosis.** The low back pain is a key symptom and the high ESR a key sign suggestive of myelomatosis in this patient. The former is caused by vertebral fracture resulting from bone destruction due to the lytic myeloma lesions. The anaemia is caused by the infiltration of the bone marrow.

4. **H. Rheumatoid arthritis.** The stiffness and swelling of the wrists and knees are suggestive of this diagnosis. The accompanying anaemia is usually normocytic and normochromic.

5. **I. Vitamin B_{12} deficiency.** This vitamin, essential for the further progression of the megaloblasts, is absorbed in the terminal ileum. The loss of this area for 6 years has caused vitamin B_{12} deficiency leading to megaloblastic anaemia. Pernicious anaemia is the term applied to B_{12} deficiency specifically due to an autoimmune destruction on the intrinsic factor producing cells in the stomach.

HAEM AND RED CELL ABNORMALITIES

11.3 For each of the following patients with a defect in haem production or erythrocyte metabolism, select the most likely diagnosis.

A   Acute intermittent porphyria
B   Autoimmune haemolytic anaemia
C   β-thalassaemia
D   Congenital erythropoietic porphyria
E   Erythropoietic protoporphyria
F   Gilbert's syndrome
G   Hereditary coproporphyria
H   Hereditary spherocytosis
I   Porphyria cutanea tarda
J   Variegate porphyria

1.   A patient presents with episodes of recurrent severe abdominal pain. On examination, she is found to have a peripheral sensory polyneuropathy and hypertension. Investigations confirm a defect of porphobilinogen synthase.

2.   A patient complains of recurrent episodes of acute bullous eruptions of the skin, especially in the summer months. A defect of protoporphyrinogen oxidase is present.

3.   A patient complains of recurrent skin eruptions on light-exposed areas that have led to scarring. The nails are also affected and there is a history of episodic confusion and sensory symptoms. There is a defect in coproporphyrinogen oxidase.

4.   A patient is noted to have a bilirubin raised at twice the upper limit of normal during an upper respiratory tract infection. All the other liver function tests are within normal limits. He tells you that other doctors have told him about this in the past and that he should not worry about it.

5.   An elderly patient is admitted by her general practitioner, complaining of shortness of breath. On examination, she looks pale, is mildly jaundiced and has moderate splenomegaly. Investigations include a haemoglobin of 5.6 and a positive Coombs' test.

Answers to 11.3

1. **A. Acute intermittent porphyria.** This is an autosomal dominant disorder but with incomplete penetrance, so other family members with the condition may never have symptoms. Attacks may be precipitated by a large number of drugs and alcohol (P450 enzyme inducers). During an acute attack, the urine turns dark on standing due to the high concentrations of ALA and PBG. The levels remain moderately raised between attacks.

2. **J. Variegate porphyria.** This is also an autosomal dominant disorder. Cutaneous fragility and photosensitivity are important features. Acute neurological attacks are common.

3. **G. Hereditary coproporphyria.** This is an autosomal recessive disorder. The uroporphyrinogen synthetase defect is expressed in erythrocytes and there are raised porphyrin levels in stool samples. In addition to acute neurological attacks, about 30% of patients experience cutaneous manifestations.

4. **F. Gilbert's syndrome.** The inheritance is thought to be autosomal dominant in this common condition, occurring in about 7% of the population. There is a modest increase in unconjugated bilirubin due to a decreased hepatic UDP-glucuronyl-transferase activity. Fasting characteristically increases the serum bilirubin level and is useful in making the diagnosis.

5. **B. Autoimmune haemolytic anaemia.** The jaundice is due to the raised bilirubin from increased red cell destruction. The enlarged spleen is the site of much of the red cell destruction.

HAEMATOLOGICAL MALIGNANCIES

11.4 **For each of the following patients, select the most likely diagnosis.**

A   Acute lymphocytic leukaemia
B   Acute myeloblastic leukaemia
C   Chronic lymphocytic leukaemia
D   Chronic myeloid leukaemia
E   Essential thrombocythaemia
F   Hodgkin's lymphoma
G   Monoclonal gammopathy of uncertain significance
H   Multiple myeloma
I   Myelofibrosis
J   Non-Hodgkin's lymphoma

1. A 30-year-old man presents with a 1-month history of lethargy, malaise and shortness of breath. On examination, he is pale and has bruising on his skin. His haemoglobin is 8.0 g/dL, white cell count 89×10^9/L, platelet count 40×10^9/L. A marrow biopsy shows >30% blast cells with Auer rods in the cytoplasm.

2. A 58-year-old woman presents with a 6-month history of tiredness, weight loss and abdominal pain. On examination, she is pale, has skin bruising and splenomegaly. Her haemoglobin is 10.5 g/dL, white cell count 118×10^9/L with immature circulating cells (5% myeloblasts). Polymerase chain reaction analysis of a bone marrow biopsy shows the presence of chimeric Abelson-BCR gene.

3. A 69-year-old man is seen at a routine pre-surgery clinic prior to a hernia repair. On examination, there are no untoward physical findings apart from the hernia. His haemoglobin is 9.8 g/dL, white cell count 30×10^9/L, platelet count 300×10^9/L. A review of his old medical notes reveals that 5 years ago his haemoglobin was 10.3 g/dL, white cell count 18×10^9/L and platelet count 350×10^9/L. Bone marrow aspirate shows an increased number of B cell precursors.

4. A 25-year-old man is seen in the clinic with a 2-month history of painless lymphadenopathy in the neck. His full blood count is normal but his ESR is 80 mm/h. A biopsy is reported as showing Reed–Sternberg cells in the lymph node.

5. An 80-year-old man is admitted to hospital following a stroke. His full blood count, urea and electrolytes are normal. He has a marginally raised serum protein and electrophoresis shows a monoclonal band. Bone marrow aspirate shows 5% plasma cells.

Answers to 11.4

1. **B. Acute myeloblastic leukaemia.** The patient is relatively young with quite a short history, making an acute leukaemia more likely than a chronic disease. The marrow shows large numbers of blast cells and the presence of Auer rods. The latter are slender, fusiform cytoplasmic inclusions that stain red with Wright–Giemsa stain and are virtually pathognomonic of acute myeloblastic anaemia.

2. **D. Chronic myeloid leukaemia.** The splenomegaly associated with this blood picture is highly suggestive of chronic myeloid leukaemia. The Abelson-BCR gene is the molecular equivalent of the Philadelphia chromosome (chromosome 22/9 translocation). The break on chromosome 22 occurs in the 'breakpoint cluster region-BCR' and the fragment of chromosome 9 that joins this area carries the Abelson oncogene. This molecular rearrangement is seen in 90% of patients with chronic myeloid leukaemia.

3. **C. Chronic lymphocytic leukaemia.** This patient has no symptoms but his peripheral blood count and bone marrow are characteristic of this disorder.

4. **F. Hodgkin's lymphoma.** Reed–Sternberg cells are characteristic of Hodgkin's lymphoma.

5. **G. Monoclonal gammopathy of uncertain significance.** There are relatively small numbers of plasma cells in the marrow and the monoclonal band is at low concentration. The patient may progress to develop myeloma or may remain stable for many years.

Dermatology

DESCRIPTIVE TERMS IN DERMATOLOGY

12.1 **For each of the following skin lesions, select the correct descriptive term.**

A   Abscess
B   Bulla
C   Ecchymosis
D   Macule
E   Nodule
F   Papule
G   Petechiae
H   Purpura
I   Pustule
J   Vesicle

1. A solid mass in the skin >0.5 cm in diameter.

2. A pin-head-sized blood lesion in the skin.

3. A circumscribed elevation of the skin, >0.5 cm in diameter and containing fluid.

4. A circumscribed elevation of the skin, <0.5 cm in diameter and containing fluid.

5. A small (<0.5 cm in diameter), flat, circumscribed area of altered colour or texture.

Answers to 12.1

1. **E. Nodule.** A papule is a solid mass in the skin <0.5 cm in diameter.

2. **G. Petechiae.** Purpura refers to areas of blood in the skin that are larger than this size. Much bigger areas, i.e. the size of a bruise, are termed ecchymosis.

3. **B. Bulla.** A vesicle is a smaller collection of fluid and a pustule is an accumulation of pus rather than clear serous fluid.

4. **J. Vesicle.**

5. **D. Macule.** A papule is a raised area of skin while a macule is flat.

WOUND DRESSINGS

12.2 Select the most appropriate dressing to match the descriptions given below.

A   Alginate
B   Biological dressing
C   Film
D   Foam
E   Hydrocolloid
F   Hydrofibres
G   Hydrogel
H   Low adherence dressing
I   Tulle dressing
J   Vacuum assisted closure

1.   A dressing that is made of knitted viscose with built-in perforations. It is minimally absorptive and can be used on dry, superficial wounds or those with minimal exudates.

2.   A dressing made of polyurethane that absorbs exudate without interacting with the wound bed. It normally has a semi-permeable backing.

3.   A highly absorbent dressing suitable for heavily exudating wounds composed of calcium salts and usually used as a flat sheet.

4.   A cotton dressing impregnated with paraffin.

5.   A dressing composed of gelatine, pectin and cellulose that absorbs exudates to form a gel.

Answers to 12.2

1. **H. Low adherence dressing.** Removal of the dressing is relatively non-traumatic, reducing damage to the underlying healing lesion.

2. **D. Foam.** This type of dressing is very useful in wounds that are producing a moderate amount of exudates.

3. **A. Alginate.** The calcium salts of alginic acid initially give the dressing a soft fibrous texture. This changes to a gel as the exudates are absorbed.

4. **I. Tulle dressing.** This traditional dressing is useful on superficial, clean wounds. The paraffin has antiseptic and soothing qualities.

5. **E. Hydrocolloid.** These dressings are said to enhance autolytic debridement of the wound.

PHOTOSENSITIVITY

12.3 **For each of the following patients with a light-induced skin rash, select the most likely diagnosis from the list given below.**

A   Chronic actinic dermatitis
B   Drug-induced photosensitivity
C   Erythropoietic protoporphyria
D   Hydroa vacuniforme
E   Pellagra
F   Polymorphic light reaction
G   Smith–Lemli–Opitz syndrome
H   Solar urticaria
I   Sunburn
J   Xeroderma pigmentosum

1.   A patient complains of an itchy, papular eruption on some, but not all, sun-exposed sites. It develops a few hours after sun exposure and lasts for around 1 week.

2.   A 7-year-old boy is taken to his general practitioner by his worried parents. Whenever he goes on holiday with them to Spain, he develops vesicles on his face. These crust over and heal, leaving small depressed scars.

3.   A 24-year-old woman says she suffers from a 'heat rash'. By this, she means that she develops intensely itchy wheals whenever she sunbathes.

4.   A 50-year-old alcoholic man has been living rough on the streets for several months and has been treated for pulmonary tuberculosis. He is noticed to have a red, scaly rash on sun-exposed areas of skin. The rash is exacerbated by re-exposure to sunlight.

5.   A 78-year-old man develops a florid eczematous rash confined to sun-exposed areas of his skin. He finds that only minimal exposure to sunlight makes the rash much worse.

Answers to 12.3

1. **F. Polymorphic light reaction.** The characteristic features of the rash are the itchy papules (flat, raised, well-circumscribed areas).

2. **D. Hydroa vacuniforme.** This is a relatively rare disorder. It tends to resolve spontaneously by adulthood.

3. **H. Solar urticaria.** Patients can mean different things when they complain of a heat rash, so a full history and examination should always be undertaken. Acute rashes are often IgE-dependent in patients with an atopic background. The differential diagnosis includes the photosensitive wheals that can arise when a person brushes against certain plants that deposit light-sensitive chemicals on the skin.

4. **E. Pellagra.** This is due to niacin deficiency. Risk factors include poor nutrition, e.g. in alcoholics and following treatment with isoniazid (for tuberculosis) and 5-fluorouracil.

5. **A. Chronic actinic dermatitis.** The names of many skin disorders are descriptive. Actinic is the term applied to light-induced skin rashes.

BLISTERS ON THE SKIN

12.4 **For each of the following patients with blistering of the skin, select the most likely diagnosis from the list given below.**

A   Bullous impetigo
B   Bullous pemphigoid
C   Dermatitis herpetiformis
D   Epidermolysis bullosa
E   Hand, foot and mouth disease
F   Lichen planus
G   Pemphigus
H   Porphyria cutanea tarda
I   Stevens–Johnson syndrome
J   Toxic epidermal necrolysis

1. An 80-year-old man has a rash that starts on his limbs but spreads to his trunk. The rash consists of large, tense blisters on an erythematous base.

2. A 65-year-old woman has flaccid, fragile blisters, superficial erosions and crusted lesions.

3. A 40-year-old man complains of intensely itchy vesicles on the extensor aspects of his elbows and knees. The rash is also present on both buttocks.

4. A 12-month-old boy has just started to crawl around. However, he has developed blisters on his knees and elbows. These heal without scarring but lesions recur.

5. A 16-month-old girl is recovering from an upper respiratory tract infection. Her parents are alarmed when the skin of her feet and hands starts peeling off in large pieces.

Answers to 12.4

1. **B. Bullous pemphigoid.** The tense, thick bullae on an erythematous base are characteristic of pemphigoid.

2. **G. Pemphigus.** The thin, fragile and easily ruptured blisters with crusts suggest pemphigus.

3. **C. Dermatitis herpetiformis.** This rash is associated with coeliac disease (gluten enteropathy), although frank malabsorption occurs only in a small proportion of patients. It responds to treatment with dapsone.

4. **D. Epidermolysis bullosa.** This is an autosomal dominant disorder. The fragile skin is easily damaged. It often presents with blisters on the knees and elbows as babies start to crawl.

5. **J. Toxic epidermal necrolysis.** This condition may occur as a drug side-effect (e.g. ampicillin) but also occasionally after staphylococcal infections. It occurs as a reaction to a variety of antigenic materials that cause a suprabasilar split in the epidermis with necrosis of much of the overlying dermis. Toxic epidermal necrolysis may be fatal and, if extensive, it should be treated as a widespread burn.

LOSS OF HAIR

12.5 For each of the following patients, select the most likely diagnosis:

A   Age-related hair loss
B   Alopecia areata
C   Alopecia totalis
D   Alopecia universalis
E   Chronic illness
F   Drug-induced hair loss
G   Hydrotic ectodermal dysplasia
H   Male-pattern baldness
I   Psoriasis
J   Tinea capitis

1.   An 18-year-old boy presents with patches of hair loss on his head. Examination of these patches shows excessive scaling with some fractured hairs. In the centre of one patch, there are two pustules.

2.   A 20-year-old student presents with a rectangular area of complete hair loss on the back of his head. The margin is well defined. A careful examination of the periphery shows some broken-off hairs.

3.   A 60-year-old man with diabetes mellitus and pernicious anaemia has complete loss of hair on his body and head. His eyebrows and eyelashes are absent. Some of his nails show multiple, dystrophic dents.

4.   A 28-year-old woman has sparse, thin, spindly hair and thin, discoloured nails with inverted edges.

5.   A 25-year-old man has hair loss along the hairline with erythematous lesions and profuse scaling. There is a reddish plaque with scaling in front of the right ear. His nails show multiple pits.

Answers to 12.5

1. **J. Tinea capitis.** This condition is caused by ringworm fungal infection of the scalp. There is excessive scaling, fracture of the hairs ('dots' on the surface), atrophy of the skin, and sometimes pustule formation with adherent yellowish crusts.

2. **B. Alopecia areata.** Alopecia areata is a localized, well-circumscribed, oval or circular loss of hair mostly affecting the scalp, though it may involve the beard, eyebrows or eyelashes. Erythema may be present in the early stages but in well-developed cases, there are no inflammatory changes. Characteristically, the peripheral areas of hair loss are studded with the diagnostic broken-off hairs called 'exclamation mark hairs'.

3. **D. Alopecia universalis.** Progressive hair loss involving the entire body, as in this patient, is termed as alopecia universalis. Alopecia may be an autoimmune disease and is sometimes associated with Hashimoto's thyroiditis, pernicious anaemia and diabetes mellitus. The hair loss becomes complete, affecting the entire body. The nails may show dystrophic changes, with the dorsal nail plate having multiple tiny depressions simulating 'hammered brass'.

4. **G. Hidrotic ectodermal dysplasia.** Epidermal and dental abnormalities are associated in two groups of ectodermal dysplasia; one of these has defective sweat glands (anhidrotic) and is transmitted through a sex-linked recessive gene. The other is autosomal dominant and associated with normal sweating (hidrotic ectodermal dysplasia). In this condition, the hair is sparse, thin and brittle and the nails are discoloured and dystrophic.

5. **I. Psoriasis.** Psoriasis of the scalp usually starts as reddish lesions on the hairline, or plaques with scales, which often occur either behind or in front of the ear. Sometimes, there is profuse scaling along the hairline when it is indistinguishable from seborrheic dermatitis. This form of psoriasis can result in hair loss.

BLISTERING SKIN LESIONS

12.6 **For each of the following scenarios, select the most likely cause for the presentation described.**

A   Bullous disease in diabetes mellitus
B   Bullous impetigo
C   Dermatitis herpetiformis
D   Erythema multiforme
E   Herpes gestationis
F   Herpes simplex
G   Herpes zoster
H   Pemphigoid
I   Pemphigus vulgaris
J   Porphyria cutanea tarda

1.   A mother brings her 14-year-old daughter with blisters scattered over her face and hands, to her general practitioner. Examination shows thin-walled blisters and pustules, and in between there are some collapsed blisters leaving behind yellowish crusts. She says that her 16-year-old son has the same problem.

2.   A 48-year-old man presents to his general practitioner with multiple lesions on his face and chest. Examination shows two thin-walled, skin-coloured bullae on his face among many ruptured ones leaving the epidermis covering a red base. He also has some reddish lesions on his buccal mucosa.

3.   A 70-year-old man presents with multiple big blisters on his arms and chest. A closer look shows mostly intact thick-walled bullae arising over erythematous skin. The oropharynx is clear.

4.   A 35-year-old man presents with multiple groups of vesicles on the face and back. He complains that these lesions are preceded by an intense burning sensation.

5.   A 40-year-old man presents with multiple, tense, skin-coloured vesicles and some ruptured ones on his face, ears, dorsum of the hands and on the fingers. He has hypertrichosis at the outer canthus. On the fingers, some of the old ulcerated vesicles have left behind scars with indurated, white papules. Examination of the nails shows some onycholysis and absent lunulae.

Answers to 12.6

1. **B. Bullous impetigo contagiosa.** Staphylococcal or streptococcal infection of the epidermis causes thin-roofed vesicles which often become crusted because of scratching. The face and hands are most commonly affected sites and the infection can spread to those in close contact. The hallmark of impetigo is honey-coloured crusting.

2. **I. Pemphigus vulgaris.** Pemphigus usually starts in the oral mucosa and later involves the skin of the face. Large, thin bullae occur usually on normal skin and on rupture leave non-healing, red erosions. The epidermis can be made to slide over the underlying dermis if lateral pressure is applied with the thumb (*Nikolsky sign*).

3. **H. Pemphigoid.** Pemphigoid involves the face much less commonly than pemphigus. Initially, the lesions often appear as urticaria, eczema or erythema and then evolve to form thick bullae. An important diagnostic feature between pemphigus and pemphigoid is that in the former the bullae arise from within the epidermis and are consequently thin and easily ruptured. In pemphigoid, on the other hand, the bullae are dermal-epidermal, thick and not easily ruptured.

4. **C. Dermatitis herpetiformis.** Erythematous papules and small haemorrhagic vesicles distributed in groups and associated with severe itching or burning sensation suggest the diagnosis. The papules, vesicles and urticarial wheals may be of variable size and shape. The vesicles may have collapsed leaving behind a denuded red base. In approximately one-fifth of patients, erythematous blotches, looking like urticarial wheals, may appear in a linear pattern with IgA deposition. In approximately two-thirds of cases, a duodenal biopsy may show the mucosal changes of gluten enteropathy, though a full malabsorption syndrome only occurs in a few patients.

5. **J. Porphyria cutanea tarda.** The clinical features described are characteristic of this condition. The white, indurated papules over the scars are called *milia* and occur in both variegate porphyria and cutanea tarda. The lesions occur on sun-exposed areas. The diagnosis is confirmed by the presence of an orange-red fluorescence of the urine when examined with a Wood's lamp. It is always worth looking at a specimen of urine from a patient suspected of having porphyria cutanea tarda, since freshly passed urine may be orange-red or brown-red.

ABNORMAL NAILS

12.7 **For each of the following descriptions, select the most likely association from the list of options below.**

A   Bronchogenic carcinoma
B   Dermatomyositis
C   Eisenmenger's syndrome
D   Hypertrophic pulmonary osteoarthropathy
E   Infective endocarditis
F   Psoriasis
G   Rheumatoid arthritis
H   The nail-patella syndrome
I   The yellow nail syndrome
J   Tuberous sclerosis

1.   A 55-year-old man presents with hoarseness of voice. His fingers show bulbous terminal digits with longitudinal and transverse curvature of the nails. The first three fingers show a brown discoloration with a yellowish tint on the fingertips and nails. There is a 2 mm callous formation on the proximal nail fold of the middle finger.

2.   A 36-year-old woman has multiple, salmon pink, erythematous papules, 2–10 mm in diameter, on her face and body. Her nails show onycholysis, pitting and multiple splinter haemorrhages.

3.   While examining a 30-year-old woman in the cardiology clinic, you notice she has clubbing of the fingers and dark blue lunulae.

4.   A 50-year-old man has lymphoedema and a right pleural effusion. His nails are stunted, thickened, excessively curved from side to side and green with a yellowish tint. The slow growth of the nails leaves uncovered fingertips beyond the stunted nails.

5.   An 18-year-old girl has grain-shaped fibromas in the periungual grooves of her nails. As you look at her face, you notice clusters of skin-coloured papules, varying from 1 to 3 mm in diameter, on the nasolabial folds.

Answers to 12.7

1. **A. Bronchogenic carcinoma.** The description given suggests that this patient has clubbing and cigarette-tar staining of the fingers, which together with a hoarse voice suggests a probable diagnosis of bronchogenic carcinoma. Staining is caused by tar from cigarettes (usually 20 or more cigarettes a day) and moisture from sweating in anxious subjects. Recurrent friction by cigarettes may cause callous formation on the dorsum of the index and middle fingers.

2. **F. Psoriasis.** The erythematous lesions mentioned suggest a diagnosis of guttate psoriasis. Pitting of the nails, ridging and onycholysis are also frequently seen in psoriasis.

3. **C. Eisenmenger's syndrome.** The normally white lunulae become darkish blue with chronic cyanosis, as would happen in Eisenmenger's syndrome. Other causes of blue lunulae are antimalarial drugs, haemochromatosis, Wilson's disease and ochronosis.

4. **I. The yellow nail syndrome.** The clinical triad consists of yellow and dystrophic nails, lymphatic abnormalities (e.g. aplasia, ectasia, lymphangitis, lymphoedema) and systemic illness (pleural effusion, bronchiectasis) or a malignancy (e.g. Hodgkin's lymphoma, melanoma).

5. **J. Tuberous sclerosis.** Periungual and subungual fibromas (Koenen's tumours) usually appear after puberty in tuberous sclerosis (epiloia). The angiofibromata seen on the nasolabial folds of this patient are pathognomonic of this condition. The principal early manifestations are the triad of seizures, mental retardation and facial angiofibromata. The presence of periungual fibromas aid the diagnosis.

SKIN LESIONS I

12.8 **For each of the following descriptions of skin lesions, select the most likely diagnosis.**

A   Acanthosis nigricans
B   Erythema multiforme
C   Erythema nodosum
D   Granuloma annulare
E   Necrobiosis lipoidica
F   Pemphigoid
G   Pemphigus
H   Pyoderma gangrenosum
I   Sweet's syndrome
J   Tuberous sclerosis

1.   Painful, palpable, blue-red nodules on the shins.

2.   Velvety thickening and pigmentation in the skin flexures.

3.   A circular, red, urticaria-like lesion with vesicles around the edges and a pale centre.

4.   Multiple, large, tense blisters occurring on erythematous skin.

5.   A shiny, atrophic and slightly yellow plaque on the shins with overlying telangiectasia.

Answers to 12.8

1. **C. Erythema nodosum.** Associated with a variety of viral and bacterial infections, drugs, sarcoidosis and inflammatory bowel disease.

2. **A. Acanthosis nigricans.** Associated with insulin resistance and diabetes.

3. **B. Erythema multiforme.** Associated with herpes simplex and mycoplasma infections and a variety of drugs including sulphonamides.

4. **F. Pemphigoid.** A relatively rare disorder seen in older patients and associated with an autoimmune attack against desmosomes.

5. **H. Pyoderma gangrenosum.** Associated with inflammatory bowel disease, HIV infection and arthritis.

SKIN LESIONS II

12.9 **For each of the following patients complaining of a skin lesion, select the most likely diagnosis.**

A   Basal cell carcinoma
B   Glomus tumour
C   Implantation dermoid cyst
D   Keratoacanthoma
E   Marjolin's ulcer
F   Paronychia
G   Pilonidal sinus
H   Sebaceous cyst
I   Sequestration dermoid cyst
J   Squamous cell carcinoma

1.   A 47-year-old woman complains of a swelling on the forehead. It has been present for several years but recently it has increased in size and become tender. On examination, there is a 4×3 cm swelling that is fluctuant and cannot be moved separately from the overlying skin.

2.   A 46-year-old woman complains of a swelling on the pulp of her right index finger. It has been present for about 1 year but she now finds it is increasingly irritating when she picks things up or does her gardening. On examination, there is a 1×0.5 cm swelling that is non-tender and cannot be moved separately from the overlying skin. There appears to be an old scar overlying the cyst.

3.   A 20-year-old man complains of a swelling in the pulp of the left ring finger. It has been present for several weeks and he says it is extremely painful if it is pressed. On examination, there is a small purple/red swelling.

4.   A 92-year-old man is noticed to have a lesion on the side of his nose with an overlying scab. He says it has been present for many years and occasionally bleeds. On examination, there is a 2×3 cm ulcer with raised edges. The edges look white but have overlying telangiectasia.

5.   A 62-year-old man presents with a lesion on the side of his nose. He says it has grown rapidly over the last 3 weeks. On examination, there is a 1 cm diameter nodule with a central crater.

Answers to 12.9

1. **H. Sebaceous cyst.** The lesion is fluctuant and this is typical of fluid-filled cysts, including sebaceous cysts. A central punctum may be present but is not mentioned in this case. Increase in size and tenderness may be due to infection or calcification in the cyst or, very rarely, malignant change.

2. **C. Implantation dermoid cyst.** The history of gardening and an overlying scar suggests a previous puncture injury. Implantation of epithelial cells into the subcutaneous tissues results in the cyst. Sequestration dermoids result from embryological rests of epithelial cells along lines of fusion (e.g. upper, outer margin of orbit).

3. **B. Glomus tumour.** The purple/red colour is due to the arteriovenous anastomoses that make up these lesions. The exquisite tenderness is characteristic of these solitary lesions that are most commonly found in the extremities and under the nails.

4. **A. Basal cell carcinoma.** These occur on sun-exposed areas and are more common in men than women. Unlike a squamous cell carcinoma, the edges are raised but not everted and there are characteristic overlying telangiectasia.

5. **D. Keratoacanthoma.** Clinically, this may appear like a squamous or basal cell carcinoma but the rapid history distinguishes the true diagnosis. More than two-thirds are on the face and most of the rest are on the arms. They resolve spontaneously but leave an unsightly scar. Very few transform into a squamous cell carcinoma.

LEG ULCERS

12.10 For each of the following patients with a leg ulcer, select the most likely diagnosis.

A   Atherosclerosis
B   Buerger's disease
C   Diabetes mellitus
D   Kaposi's sarcoma
E   Leprosy
F   Malignant melanoma
G   Sickle cell disease
H   Syphilis
I   Vasculitis
J   Venous ulcer

1.   A 38-year-old woman is seen in the dermatology clinic with several small, punched-out ulcers on the lower half of both legs. She recalls the ulcers starting as painful small bruise-coloured spots.

2.   A 62-year-old man is seen by his general practitioner with an infected foot ulcer. It is on the plantar aspect of the right foot, overlying the metatarsal heads. It is not painful and the ankle reflexes are both absent.

3.   A 36-year-old man is seen in a hospital clinic with several violaceous, well-circumscribed, raised lesions on his back. The centre of some of them is ulcerated. He has two similar lesions on his face and there is cervical lymphadenopathy.

4.   A 20-year-old woman is seen in A&E complaining of severe pain, swelling and tenderness of the right leg. The leg appears cyanosed. She says she has had similar episodes previously and that she requires opiate analgesia.

5.   A 38-year-old woman is seen in a dermatology clinic because she has noticed a 2 cm lesion on her leg that has enlarged in size over the last 2 months. It is raised, violaceous, has an irregular border and is covered by some crusted blood. There are a few enlarged lymph nodes in the groin.

Answers to 12.10

1. **I. Vasculitis.** Several of the vasculitides cause cutaneous ulceration, including polyarteritis nodosa and Wegener's granulomatosis. The inflammatory process results in small, bruise-coloured spots that subsequently break down to form well-demarcated and painful ulcers.

2. **C. Diabetes mellitus.** This is the description of a neuropathic ulcer. Leprosy and syphilis would also be associated with sensory loss but diabetes is much more common than either of these in the UK.

3. **D. Kaposi's sarcoma.** This is very rare in patients without HIV infection. Clues to the correct diagnosis include the fact that there are several lesions in multiple sites, the lymphadenopathy and the violaceous appearance. The tumour arises in the venular capillary endothelium and consists of spindle cells and small blood vessels.

4. **G. Sickle cell disease.** The woman presents with signs of an ischaemic lower limb. She is too young for atherosclerosis to be a likely cause and Buerger's disease is exceedingly rare in young women. The previous attacks and the requirement for opiate analgesia are common features in patients with sickle cell disease.

5. **F. Malignant melanoma.** The clinical scenario is typical of this diagnosis. The irregular border, violaceous appearance, recent increase in size and regional lymphadenopathy are all highly suggestive of malignant melanoma. Occasionally a benign keratoacanthoma may have similar appearances.

DERMATITIS

12.11 For each of the following patients with dermatitis, select the most appropriate diagnostic classification.

A   Allergic
B   Asteatotic
C   Atopic
D   Discoid
E   Factitious
F   Gravitational
G   Irritant
H   Localized neurodermatitis
I   Pompholyx
J   Seborrhoeic

1.   A 7-year-old boy presents to his general practitioner complaining of itching of the skin. On examination, he has eczema-type lesions with scratch marks and lichenification of the flexor surfaces of his elbows, knees, on his back and on his face.

2.   A 64-year-old man with a past history of a deep venous thrombosis complains of pigmentation and induration of the skin around both ankles.

3.   A 36-year-old woman complains of recurrent blisters on the palms of her hands and finger-tips. The lesions are very itchy and appear in hot weather.

4.   A 22-year-old woman complains of an intensely itchy patch of skin on the extensor aspect of the left forearm. On examination, the skin is thickened and excoriated.

5.   The relatives of a 92-year-old woman are concerned that her skin has deteriorated while she has been in a nursing home. The skin has a 'crazy-paving' appearance and fissures easily.

Answers to 12.11

1. **C. Atopic.** Eczema and atopic dermatitis are terms that are often used interchangeably. Characteristically the disorder starts in childhood and improves with age. There is often a family history of other atopic conditions such as asthma or hay fever.

2. **F. Gravitational.** This is also termed stasis pigmentation or dyshidrotic eczematous dermatitis. Both the pigmentation and oedema leading to induration are caused by passive venous congestion resulting from incompetent veins.

3. **I. Pompholyx.** This form of eczema is characterized by recurrent vesicles on the palms, soles and palmar surface of the fingers. The tapioca-like eruption occurs mostly on the fingers, palms and soles. The vesicles are intensely itchy. It is often made worse by heat.

4. **H. Localized neurodermatitis.** This is also termed lichen simplex chronicus (not to be confused with lichen planus). Repeated scratching or rubbing, often as a habit, results in thickened skin (lichenification) that is itchy. The condition is characterized by circumscribed lichenified plaques on the nape of the neck and the extensor surfaces of the elbows although any part of the skin may be involved.

5. **B. Asteatotic.** This is a common finding in elderly patients. Dehydration due to poor oral intake and the over-use of diuretics together with repeated washing of the skin (perhaps required because of incontinence) results in cracked skin with red fissures and slight scaling. There is diffuse involvement of the skin without identifiable borders, irregular vesiculation and lichenification.

Psychiatry

FEATURES IN SCHIZOPHRENIA

13.1 Select the term that most closely describes the observations in each of the following patients with a diagnosis of schizophrenia.

A   Affective incongruity
B   Ambivalence
C   Associative loosening
D   Autism
E   Concrete thinking
F   Echo de la pensée
G   Neologisms
H   Paranoia
I   Primary delusion
J   Secondary delusion

1.   A 20-year-old student is convinced that his thoughts are being broadcast so that everyone in the house can hear what he is thinking.

2.   A teenage girl starts giggling when telling you about how her mother died in a car accident.

3.   An 18-year-old factory worker disappears into her room for days and is overheard planning mystical adventures.

4.   A 28-year-old woman refuses to eat any food because she is sure it has been poisoned.

5.   After behaving strangely for several weeks, a young man calls together his flat-mates and apologizes, saying that he now understands it is all due to waves being beamed to him from the new digital television satellite.

Answers to 13.1

1. **F. Echo de la pensée.** This is also termed thought echo and is one of the auditory hallucinations considered as a First-Rank symptom by Schneider.

2. **A. Affective incongruity.** Thoughts and affect are disassociated. This is one of Bleuler's four 'A's.

3. **D. Autism.** This is the term applied to withdrawal from reality into an inner fantasy world. This is another one of Bleuler's four 'A's.

4. **H. Paranoia.** Although most psychiatrists would describe the patient as paranoid, an alternative answer would be that she has a persecutory delusion, i.e. a secondary delusion.

5. **I. Primary delusion.** A delusion is a fixed, false and unshakable belief. This is a primary delusion since it appears to have arisen *de novo*.

CHILD PSYCHIATRY

13.2 For each of the following scenarios, select the most likely diagnosis.

A   Asperger's syndrome
B   Attention deficit hyperactivity disorder
C   Autism
D   Depression
E   Elective mutism
F   Encopresis
G   Enuresis
H   Normal
I   Schizophrenia
J   Specific reading retardation

1.   A family are concerned about their 3-year-old boy. He is only saying a few words. Unlike their other children, he has never wanted to join in games. He was given a train set for his birthday and he seems happy just to place the trains in exactly the same position time and time again. If one of the other children moves the trains, he becomes uncontrollably angry. He is not very good at asking for the toilet.

2.   The parents and teachers of a 7-year-old boy are concerned about his behaviour at school. He is a quiet child who is happy to spend hours trying to memorize very precise, but obscure, facts. He does not play with the other children at all and may go the whole day without saying a word to anyone.

3.   A 4-year-old boy has started nursery school but, despite being shown where the toilets are, he wets himself most days.

4.   A 6-year-old girl has started nursery school. The teachers are worried that she opens her bowels in the corner of the school hall during play-time. At home, she appears generally happy and has no problems with using the toilet.

5.   A 10-year-old boy is not doing well at school. His teachers say that he just does not concentrate, rushes around without thinking of the consequences and often gets into trouble. He was recently stopped by the police for shoplifting.

Answers to 13.2

1. **C. Autism.** This is diagnosed four times more commonly in boys than girls and has an early age of onset. Key features include a reduced ability to relate to others, react to change and delayed language development. Ritualistic behaviour may be prominent.

2. **A. Asperger's syndrome.** This is a less severe form of autism, with a later onset and generally a better prognosis. IQ is normal.

3. **H. Normal.** Little boys commonly have accidents at the age of 4 especially if they start a new school, even if they have been mainly dry beforehand. Often life is just too interesting to ask for the toilet and a 4 year old may forget!

4. **F. Encopresis.** This is the deposition of a normal stool in an inappropriate place in the presence of normal bowel control. Some children with this disorder smear faeces onto the walls. There can be underlying anger, regression or fear.

5. **B. Attention deficit hyperactivity disorder.** As with autism, this is more commonly diagnosed in boys than girls. It is characterized by a short attention span, overactivity, impulsiveness and, sometimes, antisocial behaviour.

PERSONALITY DISORDERS

13.3 **Select the most appropriate personality definition for the following people.**

A   Anankastic
B   Asthenic
C   Avoidant
D   Histrionic
E   Impulsive
F   Paranoid
G   Psychopathic
H   Schizoid
I   Schizotypal
J   Suicidal

1.   A 27-year-old woman is noted to spend a great deal of time getting ready to go to work, being very careful about her make-up and hair. At work, she is considered a 'flirt' and likes being the centre of attention. However, on the occasions when men have asked her out on a date, she has become anxious and unsure what to do.

2.   A 45-year-old man is considered by others to be 'under the thumb' of his wife. However, he states that he is content and is happy for her to make all the decisions. He has failed to progress at work because his employers feel that he is too insecure to take initiatives.

3.   A 38-year-old man is arrested for rape. He feels that the police and women are 'out to get him' and that the particular woman he assaulted is making a fuss over nothing. He has a previous conviction for a 'road-rage' incident.

4.   A 22-year-old student is described as a 'loner' by his class-mates at university. They cannot recall a time when he went out socially or had a girlfriend. A few had tried to befriend him but they found him rather aloof and difficult to communicate with. Although he is considered exceedingly able academically, his course tutors are concerned about his ability to fit into the employment market.

5.   A 26-year-old man has been admitted to hospital on numerous occasions after episodes of deliberate self-harm. He is awaiting trial for reckless driving and possession of a controlled substance. His girlfriend says he can 'go off the rails' sometimes but that he is insecure and showers her with expensive presents each time she threatens to leave.

Answers to 13.3

1. **D. Histrionic.** This is also termed a narcissistic personality. There is attention seeking with a shallow and labile affect.

2. **B. Asthenic.** This is a dependent personality. There is an excessive need to be taken care of and difficulty in making everyday decisions without having others assume responsibility.

3. **G. Psychopathic.** This is also termed antisocial or sociopathic personality disorder and it can justify detention under the Mental Health Act. There is a lack of social conscience with disregard for others.

4. **H. Schizoid.** The main aspect of this personality type is social isolation. The presence of ideas of reference, odd thinking and unusual perceptions are required to use the term 'schizotypal'.

5. **E. Impulsive.** This is also termed borderline personality disorder. Key features are instability and impulsivity. There is often a fear of being abandoned.

PSYCHIATRIC DISORDERS

13.4 **For each of the following scenarios, select the most appropriate psychiatric diagnosis.**

A   Abnormal grief reaction
B   Acute stress disorder
C   Adjustment disorder
D   Agoraphobia
E   Generalized anxiety disorder
F   Normal grief reaction
G   Panic disorder
H   Post-traumatic stress disorder
I   Situational phobia
J   Social phobia

1.   A 45-year-old woman registers with a new general practitioner and asks for her repeat prescription of diazepam. She explains that she has been taking the tablets for at least 10 years for her 'nerves'. When the doctor tries to reduce the dose, she returns saying she is unable to cope. She is worried about her children at school, how she will pay the bills and whether she will lose her job. In addition, she has colicky lower abdominal pain and wonders whether she should see a specialist.

2.   A 36-year-old man has been successful at work and is promoted to a managerial post. Part of his duties include leading the team briefing every morning. He finds himself dreading this aspect of his new job and starts making excuses for being absent.

3.   A 40-year-old man moves to Wales with his company. He tries to visit family and friends in England but each time he drives across the Severn Bridge he develops palpitations and feelings of intense anxiety. He accepts that the fear is unfounded, but feels powerless to overcome it. He will not make the journey by train as he is even more worried about the Severn Tunnel.

4.   A 68-year-old woman is widowed after the sudden death of her husband. She seems very upset the first day but then copes admirably with the funeral arrangements. The day after the funeral, she is found in tears by her daughter and says she does not know how she will cope without her husband.

5.   A 52-year-old woman asks her general practitioner to refer her to hospital because she gets attacks of palpitations. During the attacks she feels her heart is pounding inside her, is sweaty and tremulous and everything 'appears distant'. The attacks can come on at any time and in any place but are most common when she is out of the house. The doctor notes that she has been fully investigated on two previous occasions for these attacks and that no physical cause has been found.

Answers to 13.4

1. **E. Generalized anxiety disorder.** The patient has a persistent, generalized excessive apprehensive expectation. The anxiety is about many events and not focused on a single concern.

2. **J. Social phobia.** The patient has a severe fear of situations in which he has to perform socially in front of other people. The underlying concern is of social humiliation.

3. **I. Situational phobia.** The patient has a fear of certain situations when he feels he is 'not in control'. In panic disorder, the symptoms are more unpredictable and not restricted to any particular set of circumstances or situations.

4. **F. Normal grief reaction.** There are no features of abnormal grief reaction (delayed onset, prolongation of reaction).

5. **G. Panic disorder.** The history is of recurrent episodes of severe anxiety that occur unpredictably. Many patients are initially investigated for cardiac or neurological disease without a physical cause being found for their symptoms.

INGESTION DISORDERS

13.5 **Select the most appropriate classification for each of the following patients that are seen by their general practitioner.**

A   Alcoholism
B   Anorexia nervosa
C   Bulimia nervosa
D   Compulsive eating
E   Drug abuse
F   Drug addiction
G   Food faddism
H   Normal
I   Pica
J   Simple obesity

1.   A 17-year-old girl with learning disabilities is reviewed in her residential home. The staff are concerned that she chews and eats her bedclothes.

2.   A 21-year-old man complains of erectile dysfunction. On examination, he appears very muscular and he admits to using steroids as part of his body-building programme. He is advised to cease taking steroids. He returns several weeks later saying that he is no better but that he has at least cut down on the use of steroids but will not stop completely.

3.   A 34-year-old teacher attends a 'Well Man' clinic. He drinks a half bottle of wine a day but no beers or spirits.

4.   A 7-year-old child is found to be significantly overweight. Genetic investigations confirm a diagnosis of Prader–Willi syndrome.

5.   A 19-year-old student is admitted to hospital feeling unwell. On examination, he is thin, has severe gingivitis and a rash on his lower limbs. His house-mates comment that he is rather odd, refuses to eat with them, and survives on the pies left in the freezer by his mother on the first day of each term.

Answers to 13.5

1. **I. Pica.** This is the persistent eating of non-foodstuffs. It is normal in toddlers, some of whom will try to eat almost anything. In older children and adults, it is most commonly seen in those with learning disabilities or autism.

2. **E. Drug abuse.** This is not drug addiction since anabolic steroids do not cause physical addiction. The man simply does not want to stop taking the drugs as he has formed the opinion that the benefits outweigh the risks.

3. **H. Normal.** Alcoholism is a difficult diagnosis to make. Although there are generally agreed limits to the amount of alcohol that may be ingested, these relate to population-based data of the risk of physical illness such as liver disease. A person may be drinking more or less than these limits and yet be causing themselves or others physical, social or psychiatric harm.

4. **D. Compulsive eating.** Patients with Prader–Willi syndrome develop massive obesity due to uncontrolled eating. There appears to be a defect in the satiety signals although the mechanism is currently not understood.

5. **G. Food faddism.** Occasional patients present with nutritional deficiency because of odd diets. This student had scurvy due to vitamin C deficiency. Sometimes the food fad starts as a seemingly innocuous predilection to a particular food or a belief in the health advantages of a certain diet.

THE 1983 MENTAL HEALTH ACT

13.6 **Select the most appropriate legal framework that could be brought to bear in each of the following circumstances arising in England and Wales.**

A   Section 135
B   Section 136
C   Section 17
D   Section 2
E   Section 3
F   Section 35
G   Section 5(2)
H   Section 5(4)
I   Section 58
J   The action is not covered by the Act

1.   A police officer finds a disturbed young female wandering the streets at night in her nightdress. She tells him that she has left home because there is a plot to murder her. She has not committed a criminal act but refuses to leave the area, saying she will be safest out of doors.

2.   An 18-year-old man is brought into hospital with a severe asthma attack. After receiving a single dose of nebulized salbutamol, he insists on going home. He is so short of breath that he can barely walk to the door but refuses all pleas to remain in hospital. Fearing for the patient's life, the A&E officer asks the nursing staff to restrain him, using the minimum force necessary.

3.   A man appears before a magistrate charged with actual bodily harm. After receiving written evidence from the police surgeon, the court orders that the man be taken to a local hospital for the purposes of obtaining a further report.

4.   A 21-year-old woman rushes around the house at all times of the day and night starting, but never finishing, odd jobs. She has applied for many credit cards and has over-spent on all of them by buying expensive presents for everyone she knows. She cannot understand why her mother is worried about her behaviour and reacts angrily when her general practitioner arrives with a psychiatrist and they insist she is taken to an Acute Psychiatry Unit for assessment.

5.   A patient with a severe depressive illness is currently an in-patient, on a voluntary basis, at a psychiatric hospital. He is happy to stay in the hospital but refuses to have electroconvulsive therapy. The consultant managing him wishes to carry out the therapy without his consent.

Answers to 13.6

1. **B. Section 136.** This Section allows a police officer who finds a person in a public place appearing to suffer from a mental disorder to take that person to a 'place of safety' for assessment.

2. **J. The action is not covered by the Act.** The 1983 Mental Health Act does not allow forceful detention for treatment of purely medical conditions.

3. **F. Section 35.** This empowers a Crown or Magistrate's Court to remand an accused person to a specific hospital for a report and lasts for 28 days. One medical practitioner must supply written or oral evidence to support the view that the patient may be suffering from a mental disorder that requires further assessment.

4. **D. Section 2.** This allows compulsory admission for assessment (which can include urgent treatment). Formally, the application is made by the nearest relative or an approved social worker and must be recommended by two medical practitioners—one a specialist and one with previous knowledge of the patient (usually the GP). If the situation demands more urgent admission, a single doctor can be relied upon under Section 4 of the Act. Section 2 lasts for 28 days but Section 4 lasts for only 72 h.

5. **I. Section 58.** This allows compulsory treatment when a consent form would normally have to be completed by the patient.

PSYCHIATRIC SYNDROMES

13.7 **For each of the following cases, select the correct eponymous psychiatric diagnosis.**

A   Capgras syndrome
B   Cotard's syndrome
C   Couvade syndrome
D   De Clérambault's syndrome
E   Ekbom's syndrome
F   Folie à deux
G   Fregoli's syndrome
H   Ganser's syndrome
I   Othello syndrome
J   Tourette's syndrome

1.   A man in prison is sent for psychiatric assessment because he has begun to give absurd and inconsistent answers to simple questions. For example, when asked the number of wheels on a car, he replies '5' and he states that 'Paris' is the capital city of England.

2.   An exasperated woman seeks the advice of her general practitioner because her husband, ever since he learnt that she was pregnant, has complained of morning sickness, back pain and abdominal swelling.

3.   A 19-year-old man with schizophrenia is admitted under the trauma team after attempting to amputate one of his own legs. When asked the reason for his actions, he replies that the leg is rotting away and needs to be removed.

4.   A 23-year-old woman comes home from work one day and throws her husband out of the house. She telephones the police because she says her real husband has been taken away and replaced by an exact double.

5.   A 36-year-old medical secretary starts to make inappropriate advances to the consultant physician for whom she works. When she is cautioned about her behaviour, she replies that he is in love with her and subsequently she begins to pester him at home with telephone calls.

Answers to 13.7

1. **H. Ganser's syndrome.** This is characterized by giving approximate or inconsistent answers to simple questions. The answers themselves reflect that the patient can understand the questions but appears to be giving a deliberately annoying response. It is often seen as a response to a stressful event.

2. **C. Couvade syndrome.** This is the experience of symptoms resembling those of pregnancy in the partners of pregnant women.

3. **B. Cotard's syndrome.** This is the delusion that part of the body is dead or rotting away (nihilistic delusion). It may occur in elderly people who are depressed.

4. **A. Capgras syndrome.** This is a delusional state in which the patient believes that a person has been replaced by an exact double.

5. **D. De Clérambault's syndrome.** This is a delusion in which patients believe that someone is in love with them (erotomania). Most commonly, it occurs in females who believe that a man (often in a powerful social position) is in love with them. The syndrome may underlie some cases in which people 'stalk' the rich and famous. It is dangerous since some patients will become angry and violent when they are rejected.

Paediatrics

PAEDIATRIC MILESTONES

14.1 Select the age by which the following features are typically observed in a healthy child.

A   12 months
B   18 months
C   2$\frac{1}{2}$ years
D   3$\frac{1}{2}$ years
E   5 years
F   6 weeks
G   9 months
H   At birth
I   Before birth
J   Within 2 days of birth

1. Draws a man with a head, arms, legs and fingers.

2. Jumps on the spot and can kick a ball.

3. Can build a tower of three or four cubes that are about the size of his hand.

4. Responds to painful stimuli.

5. Pulls up on furniture to stand.

Answers to 14.1

Normal development in children may be divided into social, hearing/speech, vision/fine motor and gross motor skills. Variation is common and it is not unusual for any given child to lag behind in one area, while being more advanced in another skill. Significant delay in multiple areas or regression should always be taken seriously, as should parental concerns.

1. **E.** 5 years.
2. **C.** 2½ years.
3. **B.** 18 months.
4. **I.** Before birth.
5. **G.** 9 months.

CONGENITAL HEART DISEASE

14.2 **For each of the clinical scenarios given below, select the most likely underlying congenital heart disease.**

A   Coarctation of the aorta
B   Fallot's tetralogy
C   Ostium primum atrial septal defect
D   Ostium secundum atrial septal defect
E   Patent ductus arteriosus
F   Pulmonary stenosis
G   Subvalvular aortic stenosis
H   Transposition of the great arteries
I   Tricuspid atresia
J   Ventricular septal defect

1.   A patient with fixed splitting of the second heart sound and an ejection systolic pulmonary murmur. The ECG shows right axis deviation and right bundle branch block.

2.   A patient with a pansystolic murmur, loudest on expiration. The ECG shows right bundle branch block with left axis deviation and an echocardiogram reveals a defect in the lower part of the atrial septum.

3.   A patient with a continuous 'machinery' murmur during both systole and diastole.

4.   A newborn infant with cyanosis that worsens rapidly in the first few days of life. Percutaneous balloon atrial septostomy provides transient relief of the cyanosis.

5.   A 4-year-old child is found to have a loud pansystolic murmur that disappears spontaneously by the time he is 7 years old.

Answers to 14.2

1. **D. Ostium secundum defect.** These lesions are relatively common. During systole, blood flows from the left atrium into the right atrium, causing increased load on the right side of the heart, explaining the right axis deviation on the ECG. Increased blood flow through the pulmonary valve may result in a pulmonary flow murmur. Pulmonary valve closure is delayed, causing fixed splitting of the second heart sound.

2. **C. Ostium primum defect.** This is rarer than an ostium secundum defect. It may interfere with mitral valve function that may be deformed, producing the murmur of mitral regurgitation. Left axis deviation may be seen on the ECG.

3. **E. Patent ductus arteriosus.** During fetal life, a connection exists between the pulmonary trunk and the aortic arch, allowing blood to bypass the non-inflated lungs. After birth, the lungs inflate, pulmonary vascular resistance falls, and the connection closes. Persistence of a patent ductus allows blood to flow from the high pressure systemic circulation (aorta) into the lower pressure pulmonary circulation, producing a continuous murmur in both systole and diastole.

4. **H. Transposition of the great arteries.** The only other cause of cyanotic congenital heart disease in the list is Fallot's tetralogy. However, atrial septostomy would not improve the cyanosis of Fallot's. It transiently improves the cyanosis in transposition by allowing mixing of the arterial and venous circulations.

5. **J. Ventricular septal defect.** This is a common lesion. A small ventricular septal defect produces a loud pansystolic murmur as blood flows from the left ventricle to the right ventricle during systole. The defect often closes spontaneously and requires no intervention unless it is large and persistent. However, patients are at increased risk of bacterial endocarditis, while the defect is patent.

FAILURE TO THRIVE

14.3 **For each of the following scenarios, select the most likely diagnosis:**

A Chronic infection
B Coeliac disease
C Cow's milk protein intolerance
D Cystic fibrosis
E Feeding mismanagement
F Growth hormone deficiency
G Hypothyroidism
H Inflammatory bowel disease
I Lactose intolerance
J Neglect

1. A 2-week-old infant is referred with a history of profuse, watery diarrhoea from the day he was born. He frequently cries without any apparent reason.

2. A 7-year-old boy is admitted to hospital with abdominal pain, bloody diarrhoea and failure to thrive. He has been admitted on two previous occasions with suspected appendicitis.

3. A short-statured, 6-year-old boy presents with loss of weight, loose stools and iron deficiency anaemia. Investigations show that his serum ferritin and folate levels are low.

4. A 9-month-old boy presents with vomiting, diarrhoea, loss of weight and eczema. Investigations show peripheral eosinophilia and a raised IgE level.

5. A 3-year-old boy is brought in with a history of repeated chest infections, loss of weight and diarrhoea. His stools are bulky and greasy.

Answers to 14.3

1. **I. Lactose intolerance.** This is an uncommon autosomal recessive condition but results in considerable misery with profuse diarrhoea as soon as milk feeds are introduced. The diagnosis is suspected from the clinical history and the response to a lactose-free diet. It can be confirmed by the measurement of brush border lactase activity.

2. **H. Inflammatory bowel disease.** This boy had Crohn's disease. Terminal ileitis may mimic acute appendicitis. If an appendicectomy is carried out, a fistula may develop between the affected small bowel and skin in the postoperative period.

3. **B. Coeliac disease.** In some cases, the onset is insidious and the manifestations become apparent in late childhood (short stature, loss of weight) or even in adult life (failure to gain weight, anaemia). Low serum ferritin and folate levels are useful pointers to the underlying malabsorption.

4. **C. Cow's milk protein intolerance.** The eosinophilia, a raised IgE level and eczema suggest the diagnosis. This suspicion can be confirmed by showing a remarkable improvement following the exclusion of cow's milk from the diet. A jejunal biopsy may show total or patchy villous atrophy and the condition can be difficult to distinguish from coeliac disease. Skin testing may reveal positive reactions to food and environmental allergens.

5. **D. Cystic fibrosis.** In this autosomal recessive condition, impaction of mucus in the ducts of the pancreas and in the bronchial and biliary trees results, respectively, in pancreatic exocrine insufficiency, chronic respiratory disease and biliary cirrhosis. The diagnosis used to be made by demonstrating a raised sodium level in the sweat but the identification of the defective gene has resulted in a more reliable molecular genetic diagnosis.

RESPIRATORY DISTRESS IN THE NEONATE

14.4 **For each of the following scenarios, select the most likely cause.**

A   Cerebral hypoxia
B   Coarctation of the aorta
C   Congenital diaphragmatic hernia
D   Meconium aspiration syndrome
E   Pneumonia
F   Pneumothorax
G   Pulmonary haemorrhage
H   Pulmonary hypoplasia
I   Tracheo-oesophageal fistula
J   Respiratory distress syndrome

1.   Two days after a full-term normal delivery, a female baby develops respiratory distress with tachypnoea and cyanosis. She is pyrexial, hypotensive and has frequent apnoeic spells. Her chest X-ray shows bilateral coarse opacities.

2.   A male infant is delivered at 32 weeks' gestation by caesarean section to a diabetic mother. After the initial resuscitation, he starts breathing but soon becomes tachypnoeic (40/min) and cyanosed. Within the hour, he develops expiratory grunting and sternal and intercostal recession.

3.   A female infant born 1 week post-term had some dark green stains on the skin and nails. The next day, she developed respiratory distress with tachypnoea, cyanosis and indrawing of the chest. She has hypoxaemia with normocarbia, metabolic acidosis and hypoglycaemia.

4.   A male full-term infant born after a normal delivery develops respiratory distress soon after his first feed. There is pooling of secretions in the tracheo-bronchial tree requiring frequent aspiration.

5.   A female infant born at 38 weeks' gestation develops respiratory distress with cyanosis at birth. Examination shows a scaphoid abdomen and the apex beat is found on the right side.

Answers to 14.4

1. **E. Pneumonia.** Pneumonia may be acquired at the time of delivery or shortly afterwards. Later onset pneumonia, as in this case, may be associated with mechanical ventilation, or aspiration through a tracheo-oesophageal fistula. The clinical impression is confirmed by culturing organisms from tracheal fluid and blood though treatment should be started immediately.

2. **J. Respiratory distress syndrome.** This used to be known as hyaline membrane disease and is caused by a deficiency of surfactant. It affects mainly pre-term infants. Maternal diabetes is one of the predisposing factors. The sternal and intercostal recession is due to reduced lung compliance. The chest X-ray shows diffuse mottling of the lung fields and, in severe cases, it progresses to a 'whiteout' with bilateral opacification of the lungs.

3. **D. Meconium aspiration syndrome.** The dark green meconium staining of the amniotic fluid and of the skin and nails, as in this infant, is found in about 9% of deliveries at term, but only a small proportion of them develop respiratory distress. In these cases, meconium is often found in the tracheal aspirate. A chest X-ray shows overinflation of the lungs and coarse, fluffy opacities.

4. **I. Tracheo-oesophageal fistula.** Recurrent inhalation of food may simply cause wheezing but often it gives rise to recurrent pneumonias and chronic inflammatory changes. The diagnosis can be made from a careful history and by observing the infant feeding. Barium swallow used to be performed to seek the anatomical abnormality although high-resolution MRI may now be used.

5. **C. Congenital diaphragmatic hernia.** Some cases of diaphragmatic hernia are detected antenatally by ultrasound but the majority present with respiratory distress either at birth or soon after. The scaphoid abdomen is due to some of the contents being in the chest cavity. If the hernia is on the left side, the apex beat is shifted to the right. Bowel sounds may be heard on auscultation of the chest.

TERMS USED IN PAEDIATRICS

14.5 For each of the situations described below, select the correct paediatric term.

A   Infant period
B   Macrosomia
C   Miscarriage
D   Neonatal period
E   Normal
F   Perinatal period
G   Postmature
H   Premature
I   Small for dates
J   Stillbirth

1.   A baby that is born after 42 weeks' gestation.

2.   The first 28 days after birth.

3.   A pregnancy that results in the delivery of a live child after 22 weeks' gestation.

4.   A pregnancy that results in the delivery of a dead child after 24 weeks' gestation.

5.   A pregnancy that results in the delivery of a baby weighing 2 kg after 38 weeks' gestation.

Answers to 14.5

1.   **G. Postmature.** Normal gestation is of 40 weeks' duration but 'post-term' is used only after 42 weeks.

2.   **D. Neonatal period.** The perinatal period refers to the first week of life. The infant period refers to the first year of life.

3.   **H. Premature.** A child born before 37 weeks' completed gestation is premature. *Note* that a premature child may also be 'small for dates'. With advances in intensive care, more of these very premature children survive.

4.   **J. Stillbirth.** Delivery of a dead child prior to 24 weeks' gestation is classified as a miscarriage.

5.   **I. Small for dates.** Race-specific standardized charts are available to determine the expected size of babies of given gestational age.

PROBLEMS IN THE PERINATAL PERIOD

14.6 For each of the following babies with a perinatal problem, select the most likely diagnosis.

A Caput
B Cephalohaematoma
C Cyanotic congenital heart disease
D Erb's palsy
E Fractured clavicle
F Hyperglycaemia
G Hypoglycaemia
H Pulmonary hypoplasia
I Respiratory distress syndrome
J Tracheo-oesophageal fistula

1. A newborn baby has a normal respiratory rate but looks cyanosed when breathing room air. On administering high volume oxygen, the baby no longer appears cyanosed.

2. A newborn baby initially appears well. However, after each feed, he becomes short of breath, 'bubbly' and cyanosed.

3. A newborn baby is delivered vaginally after a difficult second stage of labour, complicated by shoulder dystocia. On examination, there is a swelling anteriorly on the right side at the base of the neck.

4. A newborn baby is delivered vaginally after a prolonged second stage of labour. The mother is very concerned that the head looks deformed. On examination, there is a boggy swelling of the scalp that crosses the suture lines.

5. A newborn baby is delivered to a mother with diabetes. On examination, the baby appears floppy and lethargic.

Answers to 14.6

1.   **H. Pulmonary hypoplasia.** The extra oxygen in the inspired air helps to overcome the deficient pulmonary gaseous exchange. In cyanotic heart disease, increasing the inspired oxygen concentration makes no difference.

2.   **J. Tracheo-oesophageal fistula.** The diagnosis may be difficult to make and careful imaging is required to identify the site of the communication.

3.   **E. Fractured clavicle.** This is one of the more common birth injuries. The clavicle will heal and remodel without the need for internal fixation.

4.   **A. Caput.** This is the result of oedema of the scalp as the head has been squeezed through the birth canal. Although the appearance causes parental concern, it will settle spontaneously.

5.   **G. Hypoglycaemia.** The blood sugar of all babies should be checked if they appear unwell. Insulin used to treat the mother's diabetes during labour will cross the placenta and produce hypoglycaemia in the baby. Diabetes itself does occur in babies but is very unusual.

GASTROINTESTINAL DISORDERS IN CHILDREN

14.7 **For each of the following children with gastrointestinal symptoms, select the most likely diagnosis.**

A   Acute appendicitis
B   Coeliac disease
C   Cystic fibrosis
D   Hiatus hernia
E   Hirschsprung's disease
F   Intussusception
G   Lactase deficiency
H   Mesenteric adenitis
I   Pyloric stenosis
J   Volvulus

1.   A 5-week-old boy is admitted to hospital with a 2-day history of vomiting. This occurs soon after feeds, contains no bile and is forceful. On examination, the baby looks dehydrated and this is confirmed on biochemical testing, which reveals a hyponatraemic metabolic alkalosis. In between attacks, the abdomen is soft and non-tender.

2.   A 4-day-old girl is admitted to hospital with persistent vomiting since the first day of life. The vomitus contains altered blood and usually occurs after feeds and during winding. The baby appears dehydrated. The bowels have opened normally and the abdomen is soft and non-tender.

3.   A 14-year-old boy is referred to the paediatric clinic because of short stature. He had an uncomplicated full-term delivery and was of normal weight but by the time he started school he was among the smallest in his class. His appetite has always been poor and his mother comments that, despite this, he produces bulky stools that often do not flush away easily.

4.   A 9-month-old girl is sent to hospital after being seen by her general practitioner. The mother had called the doctor because the child was vomiting. When the general practitioner arrived, the girl seemed quiet and relaxed. However, during the examination she started to scream, flexed her legs and became very pale. The nappy contained loose stool and blood.

5.   A 6-year-old girl is admitted to hospital with abdominal pain. She had been well apart from symptoms of an upper respiratory tract infection the previous day. On examination, her temperature is 40°C and she looks flushed. There is intermittent periumbilical pain but no definite tenderness on palpation. The bowels have been opened normally and there has been no vomiting.

Answers to 14.7

1. **I. Pyloric stenosis.** The main differential diagnosis is of hiatus hernia. Features in favour of pyloric stenosis in this case include the forceful nature of the vomiting after meals and the time of onset—hiatus hernia usually causing symptoms in the first week of life. Pyloric stenosis occurs seven times more commonly in males than females.

2. **D. Hiatus hernia.** The vomiting has been present since birth and is not related to feeds. Pyloric stenosis (see above) is more common in first-born males, whereas there is no gender difference in hiatus hernia.

3. **B. Coeliac disease.** These are features of fat malabsorption with bulky stools. Lactase deficiency causes carbohydrate malabsorption and this more usually presents with diarrhoea. There is nothing in the history to suggest cystic fibrosis, which is another cause of fat malabsorption and failure to thrive.

4. **F. Intussusception.** The key to the correct diagnosis is the history of intermittent severe abdominal pain; the infant cried intermittently with colicky abdominal pain and is quiet and pale between the attacks. The bright red blood oozing from the intussusception is mixed with loose stools ('redcurrant jelly').

5. **H. Mesenteric adenitis.** The main differential diagnosis is acute appendicitis. However, there is no definite tenderness on palpation and no vomiting. A recent respiratory tract infection with a high fever are common features in children with mesenteric adenitis.

INFECTIOUS DISEASES IN CHILDHOOD

14.8 **Select the most likely diagnosis in each of the following children with an infectious disease.**

A   Chicken pox
B   Glandular fever
C   HIV
D   Measles
E   Pertussis
F   Roseola
G   Rubella
H   Scarlet fever
I   Slapped cheek disease
J   Tuberculosis

1.   A 14-month-old girl feels generally unwell and has a high fever for 3 days. She begins to feel better, the fever subsides but she develops a pale pink maculopapular rash on the trunk, neck and arms that lasts for a day.

2.   A 10-year-old boy complains of a sore throat and pain on swallowing. On examination, he has red spots on his palate and a 'strawberry tongue'. He then develops a fine red rash over the whole of his body that lasts for 3 days and fades by the skin shedding in fine flakes.

3.   A 4-year-old boy is playing happily in the house when his parents notice that he has a few spots on his trunk. Within an hour, he has many vesicles and a few pustules on his face, trunk, arms and thighs.

4.   A 6-year-old girl is sent home from school feeling unwell. Her mother comments that she has had a cold for a couple of days. Later that day she develops a red, slightly raised blotchy rash on her face and trunk. She has a temperature and does not want to get out of bed, preferring the bedroom curtains to be closed.

5.   A 2-year-old girl is admitted to hospital with a presumed chest infection. On examination, she is pyrexial, short of breath and has a dry cough. She is noted to have bilateral parotid swelling. Investigations confirm she is hypoxic and the chest X-ray shows hilar lymphadenopathy and pulmonary infiltrates.

Answers to 14.8

1. **F. Roseola.** Fleeting rashes in children are common as they recover from a variety of viral infections. Usually by the time the child is seen by the general practitioner, the child feels better and the rash has faded. The temperature may go up to 40°C. About 80% of cases occur before the age of 18 months. Rubella may cause a similar picture but the rash is less marked and most infections in children are subclinical.

2. **H. Scarlet fever.** The fine red rash followed by desquamation is typical. It is caused by Group A haemolytic streptococci and has become rarer, partly due to the widespread use of penicillin.

3. **A. Chicken pox.** The vesicles appear rapidly and spread down the face, trunk and proximal parts of the limbs. Although irritated by the rash, the child is otherwise generally well. The differential diagnosis is of popular urticaria (not on the list of options), which also presents with papules, vesicles and pustules, but usually mainly on the limbs.

4. **D. Measles.** Unlike chicken pox, rubella and roseola, measles is a serious disease in children, causing systemic upset. Potential complications include otitis media, pneumonia and encephalitis.

5. **C. HIV.** This child has chronic lymphocytic interstitial pneumonitis, a feature of HIV illness in childhood. The co-existent parotid swelling points to HIV rather than tuberculosis as the correct diagnosis (although patients with HIV may also have TB).

JOINT PAINS IN CHILDHOOD

14.9 **For each of the following children complaining of painful joints, select the most likely diagnosis.**

A   Bone cyst
B   Ewing's sarcoma
C   Irritable hip
D   Juvenile chronic arthritis
E   Non-accidental injury
F   Perthes' disease
G   Rickets
H   Septic hip
I   Slipped femoral epiphysis
J   Tuberculosis

1.   A 5-year-old boy is taken to his general practitioner because the parents have noticed that he has started to limp over the last 3 days. On examination, he has a low-grade pyrexia but is otherwise a well and happy child. The symptoms resolve spontaneously by the end of the week.

2.   A 5-year-old boy is seen by his general practitioner because his parents are concerned he is unwell. On examination, the child is lying in bed looking flushed and dehydrated. He cannot say what the matter is but he will not move around the bed and screams whenever his left leg is touched or the hip moved. Investigations reveal a raised white cell count and ESR.

3.   A 10-year-old girl is taken to her general practitioner because she has felt too unwell to go to school for the last week. She says all her joints ache, especially in the morning. Her mother says that she has been complaining of joint pains for the last 4 months but that she assumed this was because she was not keen on going to school. Investigations reveal a raised ESR but a normal white cell count.

4.   A 10-year-old boy is seen by his general practitioner because of pain in his right hip and a limp. He has been seen on several occasions over the last 18 months with similar complaints. A full blood count is normal but an X-ray of the hip shows a widened joint space. The symptoms do not settle, and a further X-ray the following month shows increased density of the femoral head.

5.   A 3-year-old girl is seen in A&E after falling down stairs. On examination, she has fresh bruising on her legs. X-rays shows widening of the metaphyses and irregular calcification of the epiphyseal plates of the long bones.

Answers to 14.9

1. **C. Irritable hip.** The child is too well to have a septic hip and the symptoms resolve spontaneously. The short history rules out chronic arthritis. A subacute slipped femoral epiphysis is a possibility but no X-ray findings are given. The slight temperature in an otherwise well child makes irritable hip the most likely diagnosis. Irritable hip, also termed 'transient synovitis of the hip', is the most common cause of hip pain in childhood.

2. **H. Septic hip.** The child has signs of sepsis and severe pain on movement of the hip. The diagnosis should be confirmed by aspiration of the joint.

3. **D. Juvenile chronic arthritis (Still's disease).** Pointers to the correct diagnosis include the systemic upset, symptoms worse in the morning and the raised ESR. Other features may include a swinging pyrexia, splenomegaly, lymphadenopathy and an erythematous rash. In young children, these may overshadow the relatively mild joint involvement. The differential diagnosis includes rheumatic fever.

4. **F. Perthes' disease.** The X-ray findings are typical of this disorder. The process begins with avascular necrosis of the femoral head and the X-ray may be normal at the outset. After a few weeks, the X-ray shows increasing density of the femoral head and deformity.

5. **G. Rickets.** Although less commonly seen in modern practice, rickets still occasionally occurs. The X-ray appearances of the epiphyseal plates are characteristic.

Surgical diagnosis and management

LOCAL AND REGIONAL ANAESTHESIA

15.1 **For each of the procedures listed below, select the most appropriate local or regional anaesthesia.**

A   Axillary block
B   Caudal block
C   Femoral nerve block
D   Intercostal block
E   Interscalene
F   Intrapleural block
G   Lumbar plexus bock
H   Paravertebral block
I   Penile block
J   Sciatic block

1. A child undergoing an inguinal hernia repair.

2. An elderly man with chronic lung disease who has a fractured femur and requires effective analgesia.

3. A young man who has sustained an injury to the ulnar side of his hand that requires surgery.

4. A man who requires penile surgery.

5. A woman who requires shoulder surgery.

Answers to 15.1

1. **B. Caudal block.** Most surgery of this type in children is carried out under general anaesthesia.

2. **C. Femoral nerve block.** This provides good analgesia following a femoral fracture.

3. **A. Axillary block.** Blocking the axillary nerve provides good analgesia for surgery to the ulnar side of the hand.

4. **I. Penile block.** This produces satisfactory anaesthesia for procedures that do not involve the urethra.

5. **E. Interscalene block.** This blocks C5–C7 and is suitable for shoulder surgery.

PERI-ANAL DISORDERS

15.2 For each of the scenarios described below, select the most likely diagnosis.

A   Anal fissure
B   First-degree haemorrhoids
C   Fistula-in-ano
D   Fourth-degree haemorrhoids
E   Peri-anal abscess
F   Peri-anal warts
G   Pruritus ani
H   Second-degree haemorrhoids
I   Solitary rectal ulcer syndrome
J   Third-degree haemorrhoids

1.   A 27-year-old woman complains of severe pain on passing stool, 'as if it were glass', associated with small amounts of bright red blood on the toilet paper. She denies being constipated and in fact had some diarrhoea a few days before the symptoms started.

2.   A 33-year-old man complains of a 7-day history of pain when passing stool, especially on the right side. Examination reveals a red, warm and tender area on the right buttock and rectal examination is very painful.

3.   A 48-year-old man complains of peri-anal irritation. On examination, there are numerous grape-like lesions on the anal margins and a similar lesion on the penis.

4.   A 55-year-old man complains of peri-anal irritation and itching. On examination, the peri-anal skin is lichenified with excoriation marks.

5.   A 30-year-old woman in the third trimester of her third pregnancy complains of 'piles'. She says she had a similar problem during her last pregnancy. On examination, there is a peri-anal swelling that appears to be coming from inside the anus. Gentle pressure reduces the swelling back into the anal canal, but it reappears as soon as the woman strains.

Answers to 15.2

1.   **A. Anal fissure.** *Note* that constipation is not always present and in some patients the fissure seems to appear after a diarrhoeal illness.

2.   **E. Peri-anal abscess.** This may be preceded by a history of a peri-anal fistula. Treatment is by drainage of the abscess, laying open of any fistula and intravenous antibiotics, with anaerobic coverage.

3.   **F. Peri-anal warts.** These are sexually transmitted and are relatively common. If they are extensive, immunosuppression such as occurs with HIV/AIDS should be considered as an underlying cause.

4.   **G. Pruritus ani.** The aetiology of this condition is obscure. However, recurrent scratching causes thickening (lichenification) of the skin and this itself causes further itching.

5.   **J. Third-degree haemorrhoids.** *Note* that first-degree are internal, second-degree prolapse during straining but reduce spontaneously, third-degree reduce with gentle pressure and fourth-degree are permanently prolapsed.

SUTURES, STAPLES AND LIGATURES

15.3 **A list of materials is given below. For each description that follows, select the one that most closely matches the description.**

A Catgut
B Cyanoacrylate
C Nylon
D Polyester
E Polypropylene
F Silk
G Stainless steel
H Steri-Strips®
I Titanium
J Vicryl

1. A self-adhesive tape that can be used for superficial lacerations of the face and fingers.

2. The substance from which surgical staples are produced.

3. The main component of tissue adhesives.

4. A suture material that has caused some concern because of the potential risk of transmitting prion diseases.

5. A non-absorbable suture material with no memory.

Answers to 15.3

1.   **H. Steri-Strips**®. These should not be used on deep lacerations or on those that are infected. They are particularly useful for use in children.

2.   **I. Titanium.** This is a stable, strong and inert element that is used for surgical staples and a variety of prostheses.

3.   **B. Cyanoacrylate.** Tissue adhesives or 'glues' are being increasingly used to bring lacerations into apposition. Acrylates are also the basic ingredient of household 'superglues'.

4.   **A. Catgut.** Prion diseases, such as CJD, occur in a variety of mammals and the use of materials derived from these animals carries a theoretical, potential risk of transmission.

5.   **F. Silk.** Some materials such as catgut and vicryl are broken down by the body relatively rapidly. Others, such as silk, remain for many years. 'Memory' relates to the property of a suture material to retain a previous shape. Materials with a high memory may be difficult to work with.

STOMAS

15.4 For each of the following clinical descriptions, select the most likely type of stoma from the list given below.

A Appendicostomy
B Caecostomy
C End colostomy
D End ileostomy
E Gastrostomy
F Ileal conduit
G Koch's continent ileostomy
H Loop colostomy
I Loop ileostomy
J Nephrostomy

1. An opening in the right iliac fossa fashioned after surgery for familial polyposis coli.

2. Implantation of the ureters into an isolated segment of ileum and exteriorization after a total cystectomy.

3. An opening in the left iliac fossa with a plastic rod visible, designed to divert faecal flow and protect a distal anastomosis.

4. An opening in the right iliac fossa fashioned during emergency surgery to decompress a grossly dilated colon.

5. An opening in the epigastrium fashioned in an elderly lady following a stroke.

Answers to 15.4

1. **D. End ileostomy.** The patient has had a total colectomy for polyposis coli. The terminal ileum is brought out on to the anterior abdominal wall.

2. **F. Ileal conduit.** Urine drains into the bag.

3. **I. Loop colostomy.** The plastic rod helps prevent retraction of the stoma.

4. **B. Caecostomy.** In obstruction (or pseudo-obstruction) of the large colon, the caecum distends greatly. Perfoming a caecostomy will decompress the colon and allow the wall to recover before attempting a more definitive surgery, if required.

5. **E. Gastrostomy.** A percutaneous gastrostomy is positioned with the aid of an endoscope and may be used to feed patients with unsafe swallow reflexes.

ACUTE ABDOMEN

15.5 **Put the most likely diagnosis against each abdominal catastrophe described below.**

A   Acute appendicitis
B   Acute intestinal obstruction
C   Acute pancreatitis
D   Acute porphyria
E   Mesenteric arterial thromboembolism
F   Paralytic ileus
G   Perforated peptic ulcer
H   Ruptured aortic aneurysm
I   Sigmoid colon volvulus
J   Toxic megacolon

1. A 42-year-old heavy smoker was brought to hospital 8 h after a severe upper abdominal pain. On examination, he looked toxaemic with a pulse rate of 100 bpm, and a BP of 90/50 mmHg. His abdomen looked flat and felt hard and tender on palpation.

2. A 55-year-old civil servant and habitual drinker was brought to hospital with a severe abdominal pain of 2 hours' duration. He described the pain as radiating to the back. He was restless and only derived some relief in the sitting position. He was cold and clammy with a pulse rate of 120 bpm, BP of 100/60 mmHg, and there was a bruise on his left flank.

3. A 12-year-old boy was admitted to hospital with abdominal pain of 24 hours' duration. It started like a colicky pain around the umbilicus and then settled in the right lower abdomen. He was pyrexial (38°C).

4. A 34-year-old lorry driver was brought to hospital in a collapsed state with bouts of colicky abdominal pain and incessant vomiting of 6 hours' duration. His pulse rate was 120 bpm and the systolic BP was 100 mmHg. The examination of the abdomen showed two scars of old surgery and a series of tinkling sounds through auscultation.

5. A 43-year-old nun was admitted with bouts of severe, colicky abdominal pain. Her medical history included episodes of premenstrual tension and constipation, which had become worse in the preceding week when she was started on hormone replacement therapy. Apart from a tachycardia, there were very few signs. Her abdomen was soft and the X-ray showed dilated loops of the small bowel.

Answers to 15.5

1. **G. Perforated peptic ulcer.** The sudden onset of upper abdominal pain, its severity and radiation down the flanks, the toxaemia and the board-like rigidity of the abdomen all suggest perforation leading to chemical peritonitis. It should be distinguished from an acute myocardial infarction, a leaking abdominal aneurysm and acute pancreatitis. A straight X-ray of the abdomen will show gas under the right diaphragm.

2. **C. Acute pancreatitis.** The history of long and high alcohol consumption is an aetiological factor for acute pancreatitis. The deep abdominal pain radiating to the back, jaundice and the circulatory collapse are all suggestive of this diagnosis. The bruise seen on the flank is caused by retroperitoneal haemorrhage in acute pancreatitis, and known as Grey Turner's sign.

3. **A. Acute appendicitis.** The clinical presentation of a central colicky pain, which settles down in the right iliac fossa where rebound tenderness can be elicited, is typical of this diagnosis. Pyrexia is usually mild, seldom exceeding 38°C.

4. **B. Acute intestinal obstruction.** The vomiting of copious fluids of intestinal secretions is important from both diagnostic as well as clinical standpoints, because it causes rapid dehydration, vascular collapse and electrolyte disturbance. The history of previous abdominal surgery is relevant since the resulting adhesions probably incarcerated the small intestine, causing obstruction. The gurgling and later tinkling sounds are caused by enteric fluid splashing against the resonant gas-filled intestinal walls. A straight X-ray of the abdomen will show gas and fluid levels.

5. **D. Acute porphyria.** The severity of abdominal pain is out of proportion to the abdominal findings which are usually absent; rebound tenderness is seldom present. Tachycardia is usually present and is of prognostic significance. The abdominal manifestation is believed to represent a neurogenic motility disturbance; hence the presence of dilated loops of the small intestine, a sign that may be confused with paralytic ileus. The urine will turn orange-red on standing due to the presence of uroporphyrins and porphobilinogens, which can be measured by a rapid qualitative method. A wide variety of drugs such as oestrogens, sulphonamides and chlorpropamide precipitate acute attack.

SURGICAL MANAGEMENT

15.6 **Select the most appropriate plan of action in each of the cases described below.**

A	Defer surgery for at least 1 month
B	Defer surgery for at least 6 months
C	Do not operate and discharge patient
D	Do not operate but arrange palliative care
E	Do not operate but refer to physician
F	Do not operate but review patient in surgical clinic
G	Operate immediately
H	Operate on next routine list (within 3 days)
I	Operate urgently (within 4 h)
J	Place on routine waiting list

1. A 30-year-old man has a 6-month history of persistent abnormal liver function tests for which no satisfactory cause has been found. He is admitted for a liver biopsy which is performed on the ward. You are called to review him 30 min later when he is found collapsed. His pulse is 120 bpm, his blood pressure is unrecordable and his abdomen is distended and tender.

2. An 18-year-old man is admitted in the early hours of the morning with severe pain and swelling of the scrotum. On examination, his pulse is 110 bpm, blood pressure 175/90 mmHg and he is apyrexial. The left testis is very tender and hanging high in the scrotum.

3. A 63-year-old woman is seen in the surgical clinic because of a lump in her right breast. She says it has been present for around 6 months and is non-tender. She declines to be examined further and says she does not want an operation.

4. A 41-year-old man is admitted to hospital with a 24-h history of diarrhoea and vomiting that settled spontaneously. On examination, he is noted to have a reducible left inguinal hernia. He says it has been present for over a year but has become increasingly troublesome.

5. A 44-year-old woman is admitted for a planned cholecystectomy. On admission, her blood pressure is found to be 190/100 mmHg, but it falls to the normal range when it is re-checked several times later in the day.

Answers to 15.6

1. **G. Operate immediately.** This is a life-threatening situation and there is no time to lose. He is bleeding from the liver biopsy site and this may occur even in patients with normal clotting and when the biopsy has been straightforward. Resuscitation with plasma expanders or blood should be started but, if he is bleeding briskly, he requires immediate surgery since it will not be possible to keep up with the blood loss and every moment's delay will worsen the outlook. This is one of the occasions where surgeons have been known to operate without transferring the patient to theatre.

2. **I. Operate urgently.** This man has torsion of the testis. The longer it is left, the more likely that permanent damage will result. However, it is not a life-threatening situation and there is time to complete standard preoperative surgical and anaesthetic procedures.

3. **F. Do not operate but review patient in surgical clinic.** Patients may decline to be examined or treated for many reasons, including lack of understanding, fear or some stressful event (e.g. this woman had been waiting a long time in the clinic and was anxious to pick up her children from school). It is important not to be angered by such a situation. The patient may have a breast cancer that should be treated and it would be most appropriate to send her another appointment to the surgical clinic, perhaps asking the general practitioner to speak to her as well.

4. **J. Place on routine waiting list.** The hospital admission does not appear to be related to the hernia which is an incidental finding. However, it is causing symptoms and therefore the patient may be placed on the waiting list to have it repaired. It would seem unfair to operate on the next available routine list since there is no acute problem and he would then take the place of someone who has been waiting for longer.

5. **H. Operate on next routine list.** The blood pressure is likely to have been elevated due to anxiety since it has settled spontaneously. Other reassuring features would include no hypertensive retinopathy and a normal ECG and chest X-ray.

SURGICAL PROCEDURES

15.7 For each of the following patients, select the most appropriate surgical procedure.

A   Colectomy with ileo-rectal anastomosis
B   Double-barrelled colostomy
C   End colostomy
D   Ileostomy
E   Ivor Lewis procedure
F   Loop colostomy
G   Orchidectomy
H   Orchidopexy
I   Park's pouch
J   Right hemicolectomy with primary anastomosis

1.   A 12-year-old boy with an undescended right testis lying at the inguinal ring.

2.   A patient with a Duke's stage B carcinoma of the ascending colon.

3.   A patient with a low rectal cancer requiring total rectal excision.

4.   A patient with a sigmoid volvulus that has failed to respond to the passage of a flatus tube.

5.   A patient with Crohn's disease and extensive colonic disease that has failed to respond to medical therapy.

Answers to 15.7

1. **H. Orchidopexy.** The testis should be placed in the scrotum. Even when replaced, there is an increased risk of carcinoma and the patient should be warned to report any change in size or shape in the future.

2. **J. Right hemicolectomy with primary anastomosis.** Providing there are no complicating factors, such as perforation, a single stage procedure should be performed. Despite this, patients are usually consented for a colostomy in case it proves unavoidable during the procedure.

3. **C. End colostomy.** Advances in surgical techniques have meant that fewer patients with rectal cancer require colostomy since primary anastomosis can be performed with low lying tumours. Nevertheless, some patients will require rectal excision and then the proximal colon is brought out on to the skin as an end colostomy.

4. **B. Double-barrelled colostomy.** This consists of proximal and distal colon brought out adjacent to each other, with the intervening colon removed. It is a useful procedure for the treatment of a sigmoid volvulus with a long redundant loop of sigmoid. The colostomy may be reversed at a later date.

5. **D. Ileostomy.** Many patients with inflammatory bowel disease are controlled with medical therapy. If this fails, surgical resection of the diseased bowel is required. In ulcerative colitis, total colectomy with an ileo-rectal anastomosis may be performed in an attempt to avoid the need for a stoma. In severe Crohn's disease, recurrence commonly occurs at the site of the anastomosis with sepsis and fistula formation, so a permanent ileostomy is the more usual therapeutic option.

VASCULAR SURGERY

15.8 **For each of the following clinical scenarios, select the most appropriate surgical approach.**

A	Amputation
B	Angioplasty
C	Dacron graft commencing at aortic root
D	Endarterectomy
E	Embolectomy
F	Formation of an arteriovenous fistula
G	Regular ultrasound scans
H	Surgical clipping
I	Sympathectomy
J	Thrombolysis

1. A 37-year-old man complains of sudden-onset severe headache. On examination, he has neck stiffness but no other abnormal physical signs. A CT head scan and lumbar puncture confirm a subarachnoid haemorrhage and angiography reveals aneurysms on the left middle cerebral artery and posterior communicating artery.

2. A 48-year-old man is admitted to hospital with slurred speech and weakness of his right upper limb. The following day, all his neurological signs have resolved. Physical examination is normal and he has no carotid bruits but carotid Doppler studies show an 80% stenosis at the bifurcation of the left carotid artery.

3. A 58-year-old woman is admitted complaining of shortness of breath and chest pain. Physical examination shows her to be in atrial fibrillation and all her peripheral pulses are palpable. The following day she develops severe pain in the left foot. On examination, the foot has become pale and cold and no pulses can be felt below the left femoral.

4. A 68-year-old man is being investigated for abdominal pain and abnormal liver function tests. An abdominal ultrasound reveals gallstones and a dilated common bile duct. Incidentally, a 4 cm dilatation of the abdominal aorta is reported.

5. A 75-year-old man with type 2 diabetes has suffered from intermittent claudication for several years. He has had a previous femoropopliteal bypass and angioplasties but unfortunately continues to smoke. He now presents with an ischaemic ulcer on the left great toe that is not infected but will not heal.

Answers to 15.8

1. **H. Surgical clipping.** At least 30% of patients will re-bleed and of these, half will die. The patient has no contraindications to neurosurgical intervention.

2. **D. Endarterectomy.** Patients with >70% stenosis should be considered for surgery, especially if they are symptomatic. The absence of a carotid bruit is irrelevant to the decision.

3. **B. Angioplasty.** The history is of an arterial embolus with critical ischaemia of the left foot. The embolus may be expelled by passing a Fogarty catheter into the vessel with the balloon collapsed and then drawing back with the balloon inflated.

4. **G. Regular ultrasound scans.** There is no suggestion that the aneurysm is leaking but there is a significant risk that it will increase in size in the future. Regular (yearly) scans should be performed and elective surgery considered if the aneurysm becomes >6 cm in diameter.

5. **I. Sympathectomy.** Further arterial surgery is unlikely to help this man and we are given no clinical information to suggest the presence of a specific lesion amenable to angioplasty. A sympathectomy will improve skin perfusion and may help to heal the chronic ischaemic ulcer.

BREAST DISEASE

15.9 **For each of the following patients with breast disease, select the most likely diagnosis.**

A   Breast abscess
B   Carcinoma
C   Chondroma
D   Fat necrosis
E   Fibroadenoma
F   Fibrocystic disease
G   Intraductal papilloma
H   Lipoma
I   Mammary duct ectasia
J   Tuberculous abscess

1.   A 22-year-old woman presents to her general practitioner because she has noticed a dull ache and lump in her left breast. On examination, a 3×3 cm lump can be felt in the upper medial part of the breast. It is not attached to the skin and can be easily moved around. A similar lump is found in the right breast.

2.   A 42-year-old woman presents to her general practitioner in an anxious state because she has noticed some bleeding from her right nipple. On examination, there is a 1×0.5 cm swelling adjacent to the nipple and, when pressed, blood discharges from the nipple.

3.   A 58-year-old woman is found to have a 3×4 cm lump in the upper lateral aspect of her right breast. She says the lump has been present for at least 6 months and seemed to develop after she hurt her breast with a seat belt in a road traffic accident. On examination, the nipple is inverted and the lump is attached to the overlying skin. Two small lumps can be felt in the axilla.

4.   A 17-year-old woman presents with a tender lump in her right breast. She had her nipples pierced 2 weeks previously and recalls the area becoming very red and inflamed. However, these symptoms had settled down after she took some antibiotics that she had 'left-over' from a previous visit to the general practitioner.

5.   A 40-year-old woman complains of a thick yellow/green discharge from her right nipple. She also has an occasional discharge from the left nipple. On examination, there do not appear to be any breast lumps but the nipples are retracted.

Answers to 15.9

1. **E. Fibroadenoma.** The patient is relatively young, and although carcinoma may occur at any age, it is rare under the age of 30 years. The highly mobile nature of the lump, together with the finding of a second similar lesion, suggests the diagnosis of fibroadenoma.

2. **I. Intraductal papilloma.** This is the most common cause of a blood-stained discharge from the nipple. The next most common cause is adenocarcinoma. Intraductal papillomas are not always palpable.

3. **B. Carcinoma.** It may be difficult to distinguish fat necrosis from a carcinoma without biopsy. Nipple retraction, skin tethering and even an enlarged lymph node may be present with fat necrosis. However, the correct diagnosis in this woman was carcinoma.

4. **A. Breast abscess.** These are most common in lactating women but, with the recent popularity of body piercing, other predisposing factors need to be considered. Axillary lymph nodes may be enlarged due to the infection and biopsy may be necessary to exclude malignancy and establish the true diagnosis.

5. **I. Mammary duct ectasia.** This is frequently bilateral and results from abnormal dilatation of peri-areolar lactiferous ducts. The process commences as periductal inflammation and progresses to destruction and dilatation of the ductular system. These lesions usually occur in the late pre-menopausal age group and must be distinguished from malignancy.

POSTOPERATIVE COMPLICATIONS

15.10 For each of the following patients who have recently had surgery, select the most likely postoperative complication.

A   Bronchopneumonia
B   Enterocolitis
C   Incisional hernia
D   Megaloblastic anaemia
E   Paralytic ileus
F   Pulmonary collapse
G   Pulmonary embolus
H   Reactionary haemorrhage
I   Secondary haemorrhage
J   Wound dehiscence

1.   You are asked to review an 83-year-old woman 10 days after she underwent a partial gastrectomy. She has had a stormy postoperative course and has been treated with intravenous cefotaxime for the last 5 days, as well as receiving parenteral nutrition. Over the last 24 h, she has complained of colicky lower abdominal pain and has developed profuse, offensive diarrhoea.

2.   You are called to see a 58-year-old man who underwent a colonic resection the previous day. He is short of breath. He has a 'fruity' cough but attempts at bringing up sputum are inhibited by abdominal pain. He is pyrexial and has reduced breath sounds with coarse crackles at the right base.

3.   You are called to see a 64-year-old man urgently in A&E. He had gone home earlier that week following a colonic resection performed 10 days previously. He had noticed a pink/red discharge from his abdominal wound for 2 days but after coughing that morning, he found a lump protruding from the lower part of the wound.

4.   A 70-year-old man returns to the surgical ward following a left nephrectomy performed that morning. Six hours later, you are called to see him because he looks unwell. On examination, his pulse is 120 bpm, blood pressure 60/40 mmHg but he is apyrexial and chest examination is unremarkable.

5.   A 79-year-old man is recovering from a transurethral prostatectomy. He complains of some shortness of breath and later that afternoon he is found in a collapsed state. On examination, his pulse is 130 bpm and irregular and his blood pressure is 100/60 mmHg. Examination of his chest is unremarkable but he has a raised jugular venous pressure and swelling of both legs, greater on the right.

Answers to 15.10

1. **B. Enterocolitis.** This woman has developed antibiotic-associated enterocolitis. This postoperative complication is most common in the first week after colonic surgery in patients who have received broad spectrum antibiotics such as cefotaxime.

2. **F. Pulmonary collapse.** Bronchopneumonia may supervene in patients with pulmonary collapse but, in the first 48 h after surgery, collapse due to retained secretions is most common. Treatment is physiotherapy with adequate analgesia, to allow unrestricted coughing and breathing.

3. **J. Wound dehiscence.** This typically occurs at around 10 days postoperatively. Blood-tinged discharge is an important clue that the wound may be breaking down. Incisional hernias are late complications of surgery.

4. **H. Reactionary haemorrhage.** This occurs within the first 24 h after surgery. The patient has signs of hypovolaemic shock and requires urgent resuscitation before consideration is given to re-exploring the surgical site.

5. **G. Pulmonary embolus.** The symptoms and signs of postoperative pulmonary embolus are varied. Some patients die suddenly without warning. Signs of acute right heart failure (i.e. the raised jugular venous pressure) and leg swelling are important clues to the diagnosis.

15.11 For each of the following men, who have had prostate surgery, select the most likely postoperative complication.

A   Deep vein thrombosis
B   Haemorrhage
C   Incontinence
D   Myocardial infarction
E   Pulmonary collapse
F   Pulmonary embolus
G   Retrograde ejaculation
H   TURP syndrome
I   Urethral stricture
J   Urinary tract infection

1.   A 78-year-old man is reviewed in the surgical clinic 12 months after a transurethral prostatectomy. He says that initially the results were very good but that over the last few months he has had increasing problems passing urine, with a poor stream.

2.   You are asked to review a 79-year-old man who had a transurethral prostatectomy the previous day. He has become increasingly short of breath. On examination, he is apyrexial but confused, tachypnoeic with a few crackles in the lung bases. His ECG and the chest X-ray are unchanged from admission. Biochemical analysis reveals him to be hyponatraemic with a metabolic acidosis.

3.   A 69-year-old man is reviewed 6 weeks after a transurethral prostatectomy. He is pleased with the result although he finds he has had a few accidents because his urinary stream is 'more powerful' than before. However, he is concerned about his sexual function because, although he can sustain an erection, he says it 'does not come to anything'.

4.   A 75-year-old man complains of shortness of breath 3 days after a prostatectomy. He had been recovering well but awoke in the early hours of the morning unable to breathe, with sharp left-sided chest pain. On examination, he is pyrexial, tachypnoeic, tachycardic and in pain. An ECG shows sinus tachycardia and right bundle branch block but the chest X-ray is unchanged from the one taken on admission.

5.   You are asked to review a 76-year-old man who underwent a prostatectomy the previous day. He has awoken at 3 a.m. complaining of severe shortness of breath but denies any chest pain. On examination he is cold and clammy, tachycardic and tachypnoeic. He has widespread crackles throughout his chest. An ECG shows 2 mm ST elevation in the anterior leads and a chest X-ray shows widespread interstitial shadowing.

Answers to 15.11

1.   **I. Urethral stricture.** Recurrence of symptoms after a prostatectomy may be due to failure to resect enough tissue, re-growth or malignant change. The development of bladder neck stenosis or urethral stricture following the instrumentation should also be considered.

2.   **H. TURP syndrome.** This is due to the absorption of large volumes of the fluid used to irrigate the prostatic bed after surgery. Absorption occurs through the large open veins. The patient becomes confused and hyponatraemic with signs of fluid overload.

3.   **G. Retrograde ejaculation.** This is extremely common after a TURP and patients should be warned of its development.

4.   **F. Pulmonary embolus.** The patient has sudden-onset shortness of breath with pleuritic chest pain. There is often a low-grade pyrexia that has been present for 24–36 h before the onset and may be the only clue to the presence of deep vein thrombosis. The chest X-ray and ECG may be normal, even with massive pulmonary embolus. In this case, the ECG shows signs of right-sided heart strain.

5.   **D. Myocardial infarction.** Men undergoing prostatic surgery are typically elderly and may have other disorders including ischaemic heart disease. The clinical presentation is of an acute myocardial infarction with pulmonary oedema and this is confirmed by the ST changes on the ECG. Thrombolysis is contraindicated given the recent surgery.

Obstetrics and gynaecology

CONTRACEPTION

16.1 **For each of the following, select the most appropriate method of contraception.**

A Combined oral contraceptive pill
B Condom
C Copper intrauterine device
D Levonorgestrel
G Parenteral progesterone-only contraceptive (Implanon®)
E Progesterone-only intrauterine device (Mirena®)
F Progesterone-only pill (Minipill)
H Rhythm method
I Sterilization
J Too late, nothing can be done

1. A 22-year-old student has already had two terminations of pregnancy as she forgets to take the pill. She does not have a regular partner. She has a history of pelvic inflammatory disease.

2. A 16-year-old girl wants a hormonal pill for emergency protection. She has had her first unprotected intercourse 2 days ago.

3. A 35-year-old woman, who is currently nulliparous and runs her own business, wants to defer starting a family for 1 year. She smokes 20 cigarettes a day.

4. A 30-year-old woman with poorly-controlled inflammatory bowel disease seeks reliable contraception. Her periods are heavy but she does not have any known gynaecological disease.

5. A 20-year-old woman, who is known to be positive for factor V Leiden, asks for contraception advice. She has no children but has had two terminations of pregnancy over the last 12 months. She has a poor record of attending follow-up appointments.

Answers to 16.1

1. **B. Condom.** A male or female condom would be preferable to use for this patient who has periodic sex, is not a reliable pill taker and has a history of pelvic inflammatory disease. Used according to instructions, they can prevent pregnancy in 98% of cases. An oil-based lubricant such as Vaseline should not be used with a male condom because it can cause the latex to break down. An additional advantage is that it can act as a barrier against sexually transmitted diseases. Water-based lubricants such as K-Y® jelly and spermicidal creams are safe.

2. **D. Levonorgestrel.** It is effective if the dose is taken within 72 h (preferably within 12 h) of unprotected intercourse. It can reduce the risk of pregnancy to about 1%.

3. **F. Progesterone-only pill (Minipill).** Oral progesterone-only preparations are suitable for older women (age-associated lower fertility), for heavy smokers, for those who intend to breastfeed, and for those with hypertension, valvular heart disease, diabetes mellitus and migraine. The failure rate is greater than with the combined oral contraceptive pill, but that may not be a problem in this patient who wants to start a family in the foreseeable future.

4. **E. Progesterone-only intrauterine device (Mirena®).** This is a contraceptive method of choice in women with heavy periods. In addition to the progestogenic activity, the intrauterine system itself may contribute to the contraceptive effect. There may be a reduction in blood loss.

5. **G. Parenteral progesterone-only contraceptive (Implanon®).** This is probably the best option, considering that she will not need to take any pills and will not be required to attend a regular follow-up. It provides effective contraception for up to 3 years. Barrier methods alone would be insufficient and she would be at risk of a thromboembolic event with any oestrogen-containing preparations.

HEAVY PERIODS

16.2 **For each of the following women complaining of heavy periods, select the most likely diagnosis.**

A Dysfunctional uterine bleeding
B Uterine fibroids
C Cancer of the endometrium
D Threatened miscarriage
E Polycystic ovarian disease
F Hypothyroidism
G Adenomyosis
H Pelvic inflammatory disease
I Endometrial polyp
J Coagulopathy

1. A 39-year-old woman is referred for investigation of iron deficiency anaemia. She has had regular heavy periods for several years. On examination, there is a large globular uterus. An ultrasound scan confirms a regularly enlarged uterus and a hysteroscopy is normal.

2. A 30-year-old woman complains of a 2-year history of heavy and irregular periods. On examination, a pedunculated lesion may be seen protruding from the cervical os. An ultrasound shows a very thickened endometrium.

3. A 42-year-old woman wonders whether she is approaching the menopause. She has just had very light vaginal bleeding that lasted 24 h and her previous menstrual period was about 8 weeks ago. She feels tired and irritable and has developed breast tenderness.

4. A 19-year-old woman complains of heavy regular periods. On examination she is overweight but has no hirsutism. Pelvic examination and ultrasound are normal. Initial blood test results show her to have a macrocytosis and raised serum cholesterol.

5. A 16-year-old woman is admitted to hospital from the clinic because she admits to taking 40 paracetamol tablets after missing her period. She has had unprotected intercourse in the last month. Later that day she becomes confused and develops profuse vaginal bleeding. The cervical os is closed and an ultrasound shows no products of conception. The pregnancy test is negative.

Answers to 16.2

1. **G. Adenomyosis.** This is the presence of endometrial deposits within the myometrium. The uterus is generally enlarged with no obvious fibroids.

2. **I. Endometrial polyp.** The periods are heavy and irregular (unlike in adenomyosis where they are regular). The pedunculated lesion protruding from the cervical os is an endometrial polyp, as can be confirmed histologically.

3. **D. Threatened miscarriage.** Occasionally, women who think they are menopausal are in fact pregnant and this should always be excluded before considering other diagnoses. This woman has other symptoms of pregnancy including breast tenderness.

4. **F. Hypothyroidism.** Macrocytosis and a raised cholesterol are both features of hypothyroidism which is a well-recognized cause of heavy periods.

5. **J. Coagulopathy.** This woman is not pregnant but has developed severe vaginal bleeding as a result of the coagulopathy produced by hepatic failure secondary to paracetamol overdosage.

ABSENT OR INFREQUENT PERIODS

16.3 **For each of the following women who have absent or infrequent periods, select the most likely diagnosis.**

A   Anorexia nervosa
B   Congenital imperforate hymen
C   Cushing's disease
D   Hyperprolactinaemia
E   Kallmann's syndrome
F   Panhypopituitarism
G   Polycystic ovarian syndrome
H   Pregnancy
I   Premature ovarian failure
J   Turner's syndrome

1. A 34-year-old woman presents with a 6-month history of amenorrhoea. Previously her periods had been regular and normal. Investigations show a low oestradiol and a significantly raised LH and FSH.

2. An 18-year-old woman presents with primary amenorrhoea. She is on regular thyroxine for primary hypothyroidism. On examination, she is 1.5 m tall but not underweight and has a systolic murmur at the left sternal edge. Investigations show a low oestradiol and a significantly raised LH and FSH.

3. A 19-year-old woman presents with a 1-year history of irregular periods. On examination, she is overweight and has acanthosis nigricans in the skin flexures. Investigations show a low oestradiol with a marginally raised FSH and prolactin.

4. A 15-year-old girl presents with a 3-month history of amenorrhoea. Previously her periods were generally regular. Investigations show a raised oestradiol, low LH and FSH and a raised prolactin.

5. A 17-year-old woman presents with primary amenorrhoea. On examination, she looks thin but has normal secondary sexual characteristics and fine hair on her face and back. Investigations show a low oestradiol, LH, FSH and prolactin.

Answers to 16.3

1. **I. Premature ovarian failure.** A low oestradiol in the presence of raised gonadotrophins is in keeping with premature ovarian failure or 'early menopause' (before the age of 40 years). Although many cases are idiopathic, others are associated with autoimmune endocrinopathies, infection (mumps oophoritis), irradiation or cytotoxic drugs. Laparoscopic ovarian biopsy is useful in making the diagnosis.

2. **J. Turner's syndrome.** The endocrine tests confirm ovarian failure. Hypothyroidism is associated with both Turner's syndrome and premature ovarian failure but, since the patient is 18 years old and has never had a period, Turner's syndrome is more likely. This also explains the short stature. Left-sided heart defects are seen in patients with Turner's syndrome and the systolic murmur requires further investigation.

3. **G. Polycystic ovarian syndrome.** Acanthosis nigricans is a feature of insulin resistance that is seen in polycystic ovarian syndrome.

4. **H. Pregnancy.** All women of child-bearing age should be considered pregnant until proven otherwise. Women should not be investigated for hyperprolactinaemia before a pregnancy test has been performed. *Note* that a raised prolactin may be a feature of polycystic ovarian syndrome.

5. **A. Anorexia nervosa.** This patient has hypogonadotrophic hypogonadism. Copious fine lanugo hair is a frequent finding in women with anorexia nervosa.

DISORDERS IN EARLY PREGNANCY

16.4 **Select the most likely diagnosis in each of the following women attending an early pregnancy assessment clinic.**

A   Choriocarcinoma
B   Complete miscarriage
C   Ectopic pregnancy
D   Hydatidiform mole
E   Implantation haemorrhage
F   Incomplete miscarriage
G   Inevitable miscarriage
H   Missed miscarriage
I   Phantom pregnancy
J   Threatened miscarriage

1. A 23-year-old woman had her last menstrual period 9 weeks ago and has had a positive pregnancy test. She gives a history of bleeding per vagina for the last 36 h, although it has now stopped. On examination, the cervical os is closed.

2. A 22-year-old woman had her last menstrual period 10 weeks ago and has had a positive pregnancy test. She gives a history of bleeding per vagina for the last 48 h associated with colicky lower abdominal pain. On examination, the cervical os is open.

3. A 19-year-old woman had her last menstrual period 4 weeks ago and then had light vaginal bleeding for 2 days. She feels as though she might be pregnant and indeed the pregnancy test is positive.

4. A 32-year-old woman is being treated for infertility with *in-vitro* fertilization techniques. The week after the procedure the pregnancy test is positive. She then develops severe lower abdominal pain. There is scant vaginal bleeding.

5. A 29-year-old woman presents with a history of irregular periods. Currently there is no bleeding per vagina and the cervical os is closed. An ultrasound scan reveals a fetal pole of 12 mm diameter but no fetal heart.

Answers to 16.4

1. **J. Threatened miscarriage.** An ultrasound scan should be performed to assess the size of the gestation sac, fetal pole and presence of cardiac activity and to ensure that the pregnancy lies in the uterus. Nevertheless, transient bleeding in early pregnancy is not uncommon and, given that it has ceased and the os is closed, the most likely final diagnosis is a threatened miscarriage.

2. **G. Inevitable miscarriage.** The cervical os is open and this defines the miscarriage as inevitable.

3. **E. Implantation haemorrhage.** Bleeding at about the time of the next expected period is relatively common in pregnancy and may result in uncertainty about dates or a delay in the diagnosis of pregnancy.

4. **C. Ectopic pregnancy.** Ectopic pregnancy is more common after *in-vitro* fertilization procedures. An ectopic pregnancy should always be considered when there is abdominal pain in early pregnancy.

5. **H. Missed miscarriage.** Gestational age is uncertain because of the irregular periods. However, a fetal pole of >10 mm should have visible cardiac activity on ultrasound.

VAGINAL BLEEDING DURING PREGNANCY

16.5 For each of the following women presenting with vaginal bleeding during pregnancy, select the most likely diagnosis.

A   Aspirin ingestion
B   Cervical carcinoma
C   Cervical ectropion
D   Miscarriage
E   Placental abruption
F   Type I placenta praevia
G   Type II placenta praevia
H   Type III placenta praevia
I   Type IV placenta praevia
J   Vulval varices

1.   A 30-year-old woman presents with recurrent, painless vaginal bleeding in the second half of pregnancy. The bleeding has been minor, and on examination the woman appears well with a soft, non-tender uterus. An ultrasound shows that the edge of the placenta reaches the cervical os but does not lie across it.

2.   A 32-year-old woman presents with profuse vaginal bleeding in the second half of pregnancy. On examination, she is clinically shocked but denies any pain. An ultrasound shows that the placenta lies completely across the cervical os.

3.   A 28-year-old woman complains of severe colicky abdominal pain associated with bleeding per vagina at 30 weeks' gestation. The pain has not responded to simple analgesics. On examination, the uterus is hard and tender. A cardiotocograph recording shows signs of fetal distress.

4.   A 31-year-old woman complains of post-coital bleeding in the second half of pregnancy. An ultrasound scan is normal. Pelvic examination reveals an inflamed-looking cervix composed of columnar epithelium.

5.   A 25-year-old woman presents with heavy vaginal bleeding at 12 weeks' gestation. On examination, there is lower abdominal tenderness and the cervical os is open.

Answers to 16.5

1. **G. Type II placenta praevia.** Placenta praevia is the term used to describe a low-lying placenta. It may present with painless bleeding in the second half of pregnancy. In type I placenta praevia the placenta approaches the cervical os. In type II, the edge of the placenta reaches the cervical os but does not lie across it.

2. **I. Type IV placenta praevia.** In type III (or partial) placenta praevia the placenta is partially across the cervical os and in type IV (or total) the placenta is completely across the os.

3. **E. Placental abruption.** The placental attachment to the uterine wall has been disrupted by haemorrhage. The bleeding is painful (unlike that of placenta praevia) and the uterus is hard and tender.

4. **C. Cervical ectropion.** Cervical ectropion is common in pregnancy due to the high oestrogen levels.

5. **D. Miscarriage.** The cervical os is open and this patient is having an inevitable miscarriage.

Infectious diseases

17.1 **For each of the following patients with a sexually transmitted disorder, select the most likely cause from the list below.**

A   *Candida albicans*
B   Gonorrhoea
C   Herpes virus
D   Human immunodeficiency virus
E   Human papilloma virus
F   *Molluscum contagiosum*
G   Non-specific urethritis
H   *Phthirius pubis*
I   *Sarcoptes scabei*
J   Syphilis

1.   A 34-year-old woman is found to have carcinoma of the cervix.

2.   A 23-year-old woman complains of itching of the vulva, dysuria and a white discharge.

3.   A 20-year-old man complains of dysuria and a purulent urethral discharge. Microbiological examination reveals Gram-negative cocci.

4.   A 19-year-old man attends his general practitioner because he has noticed crops of small, white, umbilicated papules that have appeared on his thighs, lower abdomen and back.

5.   A 22-year-old woman is brought into hospital after being found collapsed on the street. She has a history of drug abuse. On examination, she is found to have pubic lice.

Answers to 17.1

1. **E. Human papilloma virus.** The epidemiology of cervical cancer is that of a sexually transmitted disease. It is now recognized that particular strains of the human papilloma virus are the responsible agents. This has opened up the possibility of vaccination against the disease.

2. **A. *Candida albicans*.** Thrush is a common infection and is not always sexually transmitted since the fungus may be part of the normal vaginal flora. However, the sexual partners of those affected should be treated to prevent re-infection.

3. **B. Gonorrhoea.** This sexually transmitted disease has an incubation period of between 2 and 10 days. Women are often asymptomatic carriers but the infection may lead to pelvic inflammatory disease and infertility. The organism may infect the urethra, cervix, rectum, pharynx and conjunctiva.

4. **F. *Molluscum contagiosum*.** The lesions are white, shiny and hemispherical and grow slowly up to about 1 cm in diameter. They have a central punctum that makes them look umbilicated. They occur in children ('water warts') where they are spread by sharing towels but in adults are commonly transmitted between sexual partners. Widespread lesions are a feature of HIV disease.

5. **H. *Phthirius pubis*.** Infection is often a marker of other sexually transmitted disease. For example, this woman was involved in prostitution to fund her drug habit and was also infected with chlamydia.

TROPICAL INFECTIONS

17.2 **For each of the following patients, select the most likely diagnosis.**

A   Amoebiasis
B   Giardiasis
C   Leishmaniasis
D   Malaria
E   Marburg–Ebola disease
F   Schistosomiasis
G   Toxoplasmosis
H   Travellers' diarrhoea
I   Trypanosomiasis
J   Typhoid

1.   A 40-year-old man who had returned after a month's holiday in India has had abdominal cramps and intermittent diarrhoea with tenesmus for 2 weeks. He is now passing 5–7 motions a day with blood and mucus.

2.   A 60-year-old man presents with an ulcerated nodule of 5 cm in diameter, with raised reddish margin, on his hand. He says that it started as a 1-cm reddish swelling, became gradually bigger and broke down in the centre. He has recently returned after a long, 6-week holiday in India.

3.   A 28-year-old man developed headache, fever, abdominal pain and diarrhoea 2 weeks after returning from a 3-week travelling holiday in the Indian subcontinent. His fever is persistent and unremitting around 101°F and there are a few pinkish spots on his chest and abdomen.

4.   A 60-year-old man who has been a frequent visitor to the Middle East gives a 1-month history of intermittent abdominal cramps, increased frequency of micturition and episodes of haematuria. Examination of urine shows the presence of protein and blood.

5.   Two weeks after returning from a holiday in Africa, a 60-year-old man developed headache, backache, fever and muscle pains. These symptoms became worse over the next few days. He develops nausea, vomiting and profuse diarrhoea with blood and mucus and a maculopapular rash on the trunk.

Answers to 17.2

1. **A. Amoebiasis.** Amoebic dysentery is caused by *Entamoeba histolytica* and occurs worldwide but there is an increased incidence in tropical countries. Complications include fulminant colitis, chronic infection, severe haemorrhage and liver abscess. Diagnosis is made by the detection of cysts and trophozoites in freshly passed stools. The amoebic fluorescent antibody test is positive in a majority of patients with active colitis.

2. **C. Leishmaniasis.** Cutaneous leishmaniasis may be a single or multiple lesions and usually involves exposed areas of the skin. A typical lesion starts as an erythematous papule at the site where promastigotes are inoculated by a sandfly. The lesions persist for months before they spontaneously heal, leaving flat, hyperpigmented scars.

3. **J. Typhoid.** The key signs in this case are the persistent, unremitting fever and the so-called rose spots, which appear during the second week of the illness and are not easily visible in pigmented skin. The temperature goes up in a stepladder fashion, but once it is established it does not return to baseline unless treated.

4. **F. Schistosomiasis.** This patient's infection is most probably caused by *Schistosoma haematobium,* which invades the urinary tract but may also involve the colon. Diagnosis is confirmed by detecting *Schistosoma* eggs in urine, faeces or in the biopsy specimen from the rectum. In chronic disease, usually in older patients, granulomata develop in the lower urinary tract causing obstructive symptoms and leading to hydroureter and hydronephrosis.

5. **E. Marburg–Ebola disease.** It is also called African haemorrhagic fever and is a multisystem disease starting with acute, multiple symptoms, as in this patient. The incubation period for Ebola disease is between 3 and 18 days. Spontaneous bleeding occurs at the injection site and in any system including haematemesis, melaena and haemoptysis.

INFECTIOUS AGENTS

17.3 For each of the following scenarios, select the most likely causative organism.

A *Actinomyces israelii*
B *Coxiella brunetti*
C *Echinococcus granulosus*
D *Giardia lamblia*
E *Leptospira icterohaemorrhagiae*
F *Listeria monocytogenes*
G *Malassezia furfur*
H *Rickettsia rickettsi*
I *Salmonella typhi*
J *Treponema pertenue*

1. A 7-year-old child has recently entered the UK with his refugee parents. The family has fled a rural tropical village overcome by ethnic violence. On examination, the child has several large ulcerating papules, mainly in the skinfolds.

2. A 22-year-old student has recently returned from his elective in South America. He is admitted in a moribund state with a presumptive diagnosis of meningococcal septicaemia. On examination, he has a widespread haemorrhagic rash and hepatosplenomegaly. His friend, who had been camping with him in South America, says he also had a rash a few days before but it was mild and disappeared within 2 days.

3. A 29-year-old woman has recently returned from holiday in Spain. She visits her general practitioner because she has developed multiple pale areas on her skin. The lesions are not raised and are not itchy and are about the size of a 5 pence piece.

4. A 60-year-old man is referred to the chest clinic after a single episode of haemoptysis. He is a non-smoker and has no relevant medical history. On examination, he appears fit and well but the chest X-ray reveals a 5×6 cm lesion in the lower lobe of the right lung.

5. A 33-year-old woman has recently returned from a visit to India where she went to learn more about her family background and culture. Within a week of her return, she falls ill with headaches and muscle aches. Her general practitioner cannot find any specific abnormality but her temperature is 38°C, pulse 42 bpm and blood pressure 120/60 mmHg. She continues to deteriorate and is admitted to hospital the following week with abdominal distension and tenderness. Initially she was constipated but subsequently develops diarrhoea.

Answers to 17.3

1. **J. *Treponema pertenue*.** This child has yaws, which is a chronic granulomatous condition caused by the spirochaete. It is serologically indistinguishable from syphilis. Infection is by contact with the skin lesions that commonly occur on moist areas such as skinfolds. The central nervous and cardiovascular systems are never affected.

2. **H. *Rickettsia rickettsi*.** This patient has Rocky Mountain Spotted Fever, caused by the transmission of the causative rickettsial organism by the bite of a tick. Infection can lead to a mild illness (as that suffered by his friend) or can be rapidly fatal. Brill's disease is the term applied to a relapse of the disease years after the initial infection.

3. **G. *Malassezia furfur*.** This fungal infection is responsible for pityriasis versicolor. The lesions take the opposite colour to the underlying skin and are brown on pale skin but fail to tan, becoming pale on tanned skin.

4. **C. *Echinococcus granulosus*.** The patient has a hydatid cyst. The disease is caused by ingestion of the eggs of the dog parasite. The cysts may occur almost anywhere, causing a plethora of presentations, but hepatomegaly and obstructive jaundice are relatively common. Treatment is with albendazole and surgical removal of the cyst.

5. **I. *Salmonella typhi*.** This enteric fever is spread by the orofaecal route and is more common in areas of poor sanitation. An inappropriate bradycardia in the face of a pyrexia should suggest the diagnosis. The classic red-rose spots occur on the trunk during the second week of the illness. They fade on pressure and are easily missed, although they are more apparent on pale skin. Ciprofloxacin is the treatment of choice.

Ophthalmology

PATTERNS OF VISUAL LOSS

18.1 **For each of the following patients, who have suffered visual loss, select the most likely site of the pathological lesion.**

A   Chiasm
B   Left optic nerve in the orbit
C   Left optic radiation
D   Left optic tract
E   Left frontal cortex
F   Superior bank of striate cortex
G   Optic nerve just before the chiasm
H   Right optic radiation
I   Right optic tract
J   Right striate cortex

1.   A patient with a bitemporal hemianopia.

2.   A patient with loss of vision in the left eye only.

3.   A patient with a left-sided homonymous hemianopia.

4.   A patient with a right-sided quadrantic hemianopia.

5.   A patient with an inferior altitudinal defect.

Answers to 18.1

The optic nerves arise from the back of each eye and travel in the orbit towards the optic chiasm. At the chiasm, nasal fibres (carrying messages from the temporal field, because the temporal image would fall on the nasal half of the retina) cross, but temporal fibres do not, so the left optic tract carries impulses from the right visual field and the right optic tract carries impulses from the left visual field. The fibres maintain their spatial orientation, so that messages from the upper visual field are carried in the lower part of the tract ands those from the lower fields are carried superiorly. After the lateral geniculate nucleus, the optic radiation takes the lower fibres through the temporal lobe to the occipital cortex and the upper fibres pass through the parietal cortex to the occipital cortex.

1. **A. Chiasm.** This typically occurs in a patient with a pituitary tumour. The enlarged pituitary presses on the optic chiasm and disrupts the central fibres that are crossing from the nasal portions of each optic nerve. As noted above, the nasal part on the retina corresponds to the temporal visual field.

2. **B. Left optic nerve in the orbit.** Uniocular visual loss is due to a local problem in the eye or orbit.

3. **I. Right optic tract.**

4. **C. Left optic radiation.**

5. **F. Superior bank of striate cortex.** This contains the fibres from the inferior visual fields.

ACUTE RED EYE

18.2 **For each of the following patients complaining of a red eye, select the most likely diagnosis.**

A   Acute anterior uveitis
B   Acute glaucoma
C   Blepharitis
D   Episcleritis
E   Foreign body
F   Herpes simplex conjunctivitis
G   Keratitis
H   Staphylococcal conjunctivitis
I   Subconjunctival haemorrhage
J   Trachoma

1. An 81-year-old man is admitted to hospital with nausea and vomiting. On examination, the right eye looks red and the pupil is dilated, fixed and oval in shape. He complains of severe pain around the eye and says that, when he looks at bright objects, he sees rings of light around them.

2. A 30-year-old woman seeks the advice of her general practitioner because she has developed a streak of bright red blood in her left eye. She noticed it on looking in the mirror. The eye is not painful and her vision is unaffected.

3. A 40-year-old woman complains of a painful red eye with reduced vision. On examination, the patient dislikes bright light and the eye is red, especially around the cornea. The pupil is small and fixed.

4. A 66-year-old woman complains of pain in the right eye. She noticed the pain when she awoke in the morning and, when looking in the mirror, found her eye looked red. On examination, there is a localized area of inflammation midway between the edge of the iris and outer canthus of the eye.

5. A 23-year-old man complains of a painful, 'gritty' eye. The symptoms came on over about half-an-hour while he was at work and have persisted all afternoon. On examination, the eye is red but the pupil is normal and vision is not impaired.

Answers to 18.2

1. **B. Acute glaucoma.** The pain is severe and may be associated with nausea and vomiting. Unlike in keratitis or conjunctival disorders, the pupil is fixed and dilated. Anterior uveitis would produce a small pupil. Halos of rainbow-coloured light around objects are characteristic in acute glaucoma.

2. **I. Subconjunctival haemorrhage.** This may be a sign of an anterior cranial fossa fracture or may be precipitated by severe coughing or strangulation. The history in this case suggests a spontaneous haemorrhage that will resolve spontaneously and requires no further intervention.

3. **A. Acute anterior uveitis.** Circumcorneal injection is seen in uveitis but can also be seen with acute glaucoma. However, in this case, the pupil is small and fixed; a feature of uveitis.

4. **D. Episcleritis.** This woman has localized inflammation of the sclera.

5. **E. Foreign body.** Grittiness of the eye should suggest the presence of a foreign body. As in this case, there may not be a history of trauma or a foreign body entering the eye but the symptoms come on quickly and persist. It is the most likely diagnosis in an otherwise well, young patient presenting with uniocular symptoms.

ACUTE OPHTHALMIC DISORDERS

18.3 Match the most likely diagnosis from the list against each of the following presentations.

A   Acanthamoeba keratitis
B   Acute congestive glaucoma
C   Acute conjunctivitis
D   Acute iridocyclitis
E   Acute purulent keratitis
F   Acute scleritis
G   Hypopyon ulcer
H   Migraine
I   Punctate keratitis
J   Retrobulbar neuritis

1. A 60-year-old woman presented with a disabling headache, vomiting and blurring of vision, all of 4 hours' duration. She complains of seeing a peculiar halo around the lights. She feels intense pain in her right eye that is congested with oedema of the lids and conjunctiva. The pupil is dilated and unresponsive to light and accommodation.

2. A 45-year-old landscape gardener presents with a pain and watery discharge in his left eye. The eye looks red with marked circumcorneal injection, muddy and oedematous iris, and contracted and sluggishly reactive pupil.

3. A 15-year-old boy presents with congested eyes. When he woke up in the morning, he had difficulty in opening his eyes because his eyelids were sealed and crusted. His conjunctiva are congested, there is a mucopurulent discharge, and the pupils are normal and reactive.

4. A 10-year-old girl presents with a severe painful right eye, lacrimation and photophobia. The lateral limbus looks congested. She has marked blepharospasm and pain.

5. A 26-year-old engineer presents with a painful right eye. He wears contact lenses and is always careful in washing them with saline before and after use. He has marked blepharospasm but, when this is overcome, one can see a whitish area on the upper half of the cornea. The bulbar conjunctiva is congested and there is a watery discharge.

Answers to 18.3

1. **B. Acute congestive glaucoma.** A sudden onset of headache and vomiting with a congested eye is highly suggestive of an acute attack of close-angle glaucoma. It can be mistaken for migraine in which the headache may be preceded by the patient's seeing a zig-zag pattern of lights. The pupil is dilated, oval and unreactive. The vision is impaired and it can worsen unless urgently treated.

2. **D. Acute iridocyclitis.** Like acute glaucoma, there is injection round the cornea but in this condition, the iris is swollen and yellowish green; the so-called 'muddy iris'. The pupil is small but responsive. The discharge is lacrimal and not mucopurulent as in conjunctivitis.

3. **C. Acute conjunctivitis.** The injection is superficial and the media are clear in acute conjunctivitis. Unlike iritis, the discharge is mucopurulent and sticky. The pupil is normal and reactive and the vision is unaffected. The onset is gradual and there is some discomfort but not acute pain.

4. **E. Acute purulent keratitis.** The cornea is exquisitely sensitive and any abrasion or ulcer on it causes intense pain, lacrimation and blepharospasm.

5. **A. Acanthamoeba keratitis.** Unfortunately, the saline washing solution is the source of this ubiquitous organism, which can cause keratitis with devastating results unless diagnosed and treated early. The whitish appearance is due to lymphoid cell infiltration at the site of invasion.

LOSS OF VISION

18.4 **For each of the following patients presenting with visual loss, select the most likely cause.**

A Amaurosis fugax
B Chloroquine amblyopia
C Diabetic retinopathy
D Hypertensive retinopathy
E Methyl alcohol amblyopia
F Quinine amblyopia
G Retinal vein occlusion
H Secondary optic atrophy
I Senile macular degeneration
J Tobacco amblyopia

1. A 58-year-old unemployed man, who has been sleeping rough and has a history of alcohol abuse, is brought to hospital in a semi-comatose state. His friend who came with him says that he smokes and drinks, has poor vision, and has an occasional binge, but this time it was followed by vomiting, giddiness and a steady loss of consciousness. He is unconscious but responds to painful stimuli. His fundi show pale discs.

2. A 38-year-old woman has systemic lupus erythematosus that has been stable on treatment. However, she has noticed a steady deterioration in her distant vision for the last 3 months. On examination, her visual acuity is 6/60 in both eyes and fundoscopy shows pigmentary clumping and attenuated vessels.

3. A 65-year-old retired housekeeper with ischaemic heart disease developed painful cramps in her legs after she had been treated for an episode of congestive heart failure. Her doctor continued with the diuretics but gave her some tablets for her cramps. She now presents with impaired hearing and vision. Her pupils are dilated and fundoscopy shows pale discs.

4. A 78-year-old man with type 2 diabetes mellitus on oral hypoglycaemic agents has noticed a progressive deterioration of vision for the last 6 months. Fundoscopy shows no haemorrhages but greyish maculae with a cluster of whitish spots in them.

5. A 57-year-old man is referred with a sudden loss of vision in his right eye. He says that while he was walking, he suddenly thought that there was something wrong with his sight. He closed his right eye and he could see everything but when he closed his left eye, it was all black. He can now see with both his eyes and his visual acuity is normal. His heart is in atrial fibrillation and there is no other abnormality.

Answers to 18.4

1. **E. Methyl alcohol amblyopia.** This patient with a history of alcohol abuse and binges is probably ingesting methanol which causes metabolic acidosis and visual loss. The visual loss is irreversible once optic atrophy has developed as in this case.

2. **B. Chloroquine amblyopia.** This patient is probably on long-term chloroquine for her systemic lupus erythematosus. Visual loss appears in some patients after prolonged administration of chloroquine in doses exceeding 250 mg/day. The drug binds to pigmented tissues with formation of pigment clumps, often in a target-like or bull's-eye pattern in the fovea.

3. **F. Quinine amblyopia.** This drug is empirically used for cramps and susceptible individuals can lose hearing and vision even after small doses. Blindness, dizziness and hearing loss may develop suddenly. The retinal vessels become narrow and optic atrophy ensues. Central vision may improve in time.

4. **I. Senile macular degeneration.** This patient's fundi do not show any evidence of diabetic retinopathy, and his loss of vision is most probably due to senile macular degeneration. This is a progressive condition causing loss of vision. Initially, the macula shows greyish discoloration and gradually punctate whitish spots appear in the fovea.

5. **A. Amaurosis fugax.** Unilateral loss of vision which recovers is a form of a transient ischaemic attack, caused by a fibrin or a cholesterol crystal detached from a plaque in the carotids and lodged in the retinal arterioles, or a small thrombus fired from within the left atrium in a patient with atrial fibrillation. This phenomenon may be visible on fundoscopy but often there is no abnormality after the episode has passed. Doppler and echo studies will be required to explore the cause of the thromboembolism.

Clinical pharmacology

CYTOTOXIC AGENTS

19.1 **For each of the cytotoxic agents given below, select the correct classification from the list given.**

A   Alkylating agent
B   Angiogenesis inhibitor
C   Anti-metabolite
D   Anti-tumour antibiotic
E   Cytokine
F   Hormonal therapy
G   Mitotic inhibitor
H   Monoclonal antibody
I   Radioisotope
J   Signal transduction inhibitor

1. Vincristine.

2. Interleukin 2.

3. Cyproterone acetate.

4. Doxorubicin.

5. Cisplatin.

Answers to 19.1

1. **G. Mitotic inhibitor.** Vincristine is a vinca alkaloid. It binds to tubulin dimmers, preventing their assembly into microtubules and hence inhibiting mitosis.

2. **E. Cytokine.** Interleukin 2 is a T-cell growth factor that stimulates the production of lymphokine activated killer cells. It is used in the treatment of renal cell carcinoma and melanoma.

3. **F. Hormonal therapy.** Cyproterone acetate is an anti-androgen that has a role in the treatment of androgen-sensitive tumours such as prostatic cancer. It has also been used in the treatment of male hypersexuality ('chemical castration') and polycystic ovarian syndrome.

4. **D. Anti-tumour antibiotic.** Some antibiotics such as bleomycin and doxorubicin have anti-tumour activity. Doxorubicin intercalates between base pairs of DNA, inhibits RNA and DNA polymerase, generates free radicals and alters membrane function.

5. **A. Alkylating agent.** These cross-link DNA. Cisplatin is a powerful cytotoxic but unfortunately may also have severe side-effects.

ACRONYMS IN MEDICAL TRIALS

19.2 **For each of the following descriptions of clinical trials, select the correct acronym.**

A   4S
B   CARDS
C   CONSENSUS
D   GUSTO
E   HOPE
F   HOT
G   LIPID
H   SAVE
I   UKPDS
J   WOSCOPS

1. A study that demonstrated the value of lowering the diastolic blood pressure below 90 mmHg.

2. A study that demonstrated the value of tight glycaemic control in patients with type 2 diabetes mellitus.

3. A study that evaluated the use of atorvastatin for the primary prevention of cardiovascular events in patients with type 2 diabetes mellitus without pre-existing elevated LDL-cholesterol levels.

4. A study that demonstrated the benefit of simvastatin treatment in patients with known coronary artery disease and a raised serum cholesterol.

5. A study that demonstrated the benefit of treatment with ramipril in the prevention of strokes in patients with known vascular disease or diabetes mellitus.

Answers to 19.2

There are hundreds of acronyms for clinical trials. Although they can act as useful shorthand for clinical studies, there is increasing disquiet about their proliferation. First, some acronyms are clearly a marketing strategy rather than being designed to give information about the trial (explaining many 'positive' sounding trials such as HOPE, ASPIRE, PROMISE, EPIC and CURE). Second, some are only produced by tortuous convolution of the study title or aims (AIMS – another acronym!). Finally, the same acronym may be used for several different trials (e.g. HEART). Students are encouraged not to use an acronym, or be impressed by it, unless they have read the original paper. However, this question lists some that are commonly encountered.

1. **F. HOT = Hypertension Optimal Control.** It is now well established that anti-hypertensive treatment should aim to lower the blood pressure by as much as possible rather than accepting a diastolic of 90 mmHg as the arbitrary measure of therapeutic success.

2. **I. UKPDS = United Kingdom Prospective Diabetes Study.** This was a long-term study of people with type 2 diabetes that included several interventions. It was the first study to show that tight glycaemic control reduces the risk of microvascular complications.

3. **B. CARDS = Collaborative AtoRvastatin Diabetes Study.** This trial randomized people with diabetes and at least one other coronary artery disease risk factor but without markedly elevated LDL-cholesterol levels to receive atorvastatin or placebo. Several other studies have confirmed the value of reducing serum cholesterol with statins in people with diabetes, even if their pre-treatment levels are in the traditional normal range. Almost all people with type 2 diabetes should be prescribed a statin.

4. **A. 4S = Scandinavian Simvastatin Survival Study.** This was the first major study that demonstrated the value of reducing serum cholesterol in patients with statin therapy.

5. **E. HOPE = Heart Outcomes Prevention Evaluation.** In this trial, 9297 patients with vascular disease or diabetes plus an additional risk factor were randomized to receive ramipril 10 mg, vitamin E or both. Ramipril, but not vitamin E, reduced the risk of stroke by around 30% after a mean of 4.5 years' treatment.

ADVERSE EFFECTS ON ANTICONVULSANT MEDICATION

19.3 **For each of the following patients with epilepsy and complaining of an adverse drug reaction, select the most likely culprit from the list.**

A   Carbamazepine
B   Clobazam
C   Clonazepam
D   Gabapentin
E   Lamotrigine
F   Oxcarbazepine
G   Phenytoin
H   Sodium valproate
I   Tiagabine
J   Vigabatrin

1.   A patient complaining of gum hypertrophy and hirsutism.

2.   A patient complaining of gynaecomastia.

3.   A patient with a visual field defect.

4.   A patient with weight loss.

5.   A patient complaining of recurrent and vivid nightmares.

Answers to 19.3

1. **G. Phenytoin.** The gum hypertrophy is worse in patients with co-existent gingivitis and regular brushing of the teeth and gums should be recommended.

2. **H. Sodium valproate.** In addition to the gynaecomastia, valproate is thought to inhibit the neurological development of the developing fetus and its use in pregnancy should be avoided.

3. **J. Vigabatrin.**

4. **F. Oxcarbazepine.** A number of neuroactive compounds have been investigated as possible treatments for obesity.

5. **D. Gabapentin.** This drug is also used for neuropathic pain, often in high doses. Sudden discontinuation may cause fits.

PRACTICAL PRESCRIBING

19.4 **For each of the following drugs, select the correct statement from the list given below.**

A   Can be purchased without a prescription in a pharmacy
B   Can be purchased without a prescription over the counter in any shop
C   Can only be prescribed by a hospital consultant
D   Can only be used by patients in hospital
E   Is a controlled drug
F   Is available on the NHS only to selected patients
G   Is not available legally in the UK
H   Must never be prescribed to any patient
I   Must never be used in pregnancy
J   Must never be used in patients with renal failure

1.   Cod-liver oil capsules.

2.   Codeine phosphate 60 mg tablets.

3.   Clotrimazole, 1% cream.

4.   Cannabis resin.

5.   Viagra 50 mg tablets.

Answers to 19.4

1. **B. Can be purchased without a prescription over the counter in any shop.** Many vitamin and 'herbal remedies' are freely available and their use should be investigated when taking a full drug history from patients.

2. **E. Is a controlled drug.** The prescription must adhere to specific standards, including stating the dose in words and figures and stating the total dose to be supplied. Smaller doses of codeine and codeine/paracetamol preparations are not controlled.

3. **A. Can be purchased without a prescription in a pharmacy.** Some drugs, including clotrimazole for genital thrush, can be purchased without a prescription, but only from a qualified pharmacist. If a supermarket has a pharmacy department on site, it can still not sell the product unless a qualified pharmacist is on duty and has supplied the product.

4. **G. Is not available legally in the UK.** Cannabis is illegal in the UK. A few clinical trials have used cannabis-derived medication, but never in the form of the resin.

5. **F. Is available on the NHS only to selected patients.** Viagra may be prescribed on the NHS to men with specific disorders such as erectile dysfunction related to diabetes or previous prostate surgery. If the man does not fulfil these criteria, it still may be prescribed but only on a private prescription.

POISONING I

19.5 **For each of the following scenarios, select the most likely agent responsible for the poisoning.**

A   Carbon monoxide
B   Cyanide
C   Digoxin
D   Ethylene glycol
E   Iron
F   Lead
G   Mercury
H   Opioids
I   Paracetamol
J   Salicylates

1.   A 30-year-old woman is admitted to hospital in a confused state. She complains of ringing in her ears. She is hyperventilating and has a respiratory alkalosis.

2.   A 23-year-old woman is found collapsed in a public toilet. She has been vomiting. On examination, she has pin-point pupils, is bradycardic with a low blood pressure and a depressed respiratory rate.

3.   A 19-year-old woman is admitted to hospital complaining of nausea and vomiting. On examination, she is mildly icteric and is tender in the right upper quadrant.

4.   A 46-year-old man is referred to hospital with chronic colicky lower abdominal pain and constipation. On examination, he has a blue discoloration of his gums.

5.   A 29-year-old man is brought into casualty by the police, apparently having been found drunk in the street. He has been vomiting. Shortly after admission, he develops focal seizures and decreased conscious level. On examination, he has nystagmus and ophthalmoplegia.

Answers to 19.5

1. **J. Salicylates.** These are the typical features of a moderately severe aspirin overdose. Renal failure may supervene.

2. **H. Opioids.** Pin-point pupils (not just small!) and respiratory depression should always suggest opiate ingestion. Diamorphine (heroin) is the commonly abused opioid that can be injected (main-lining) or inhaled (chasing the dragon). A specific antagonist such as naloxone may be given. The improvement may be short-lived and so repeated doses or an infusion may be necessary.

3. **I. Paracetamol.** Early features can include nausea and vomiting. By the time icterus is obvious, extensive hepatocellular damage has occurred. Treatment with N-acetylcysteine will protect the liver from further damage. It can be given even if the overdose was many hours previously.

4. **F. Lead.** Chronic poisoning with lead is now uncommon in the UK due to strict health and safety procedures such as better ventilation of factories that use lead-based products and the banning of lead additives in paint. Foot drop or wrist drop is a classical feature of lead poisoning, due to an associated primary motor neuropathy.

5. **D. Ethylene glycol.** This is the main active ingredient of antifreeze. It may be drunk deliberately or added to illegally produced spirits.

POISONING 2

19.6 For each of the following scenarios, select the most likely cause.

A   Amphetamines
B   Carbon monoxide
C   Chlorpromazine
D   Chlorpropamide
E   Ethanol
F   Opiates
G   Organophosphates
H   Paracetamol
I   Salbutamol
J   Salicylates

1. A 65-year-old man was found unconscious in a bush with multiple scratch marks on his body. He is unrousable but there are no lateralizing neurological signs. He is profusely sweaty, producing a wet imprint on the sheet under him. His pulse is 90 bpm, respiration 25/min, BP of 120/70 mmHg, temperature of 38°F, blood glucose of 8 mmol/L and his arterial blood pH is 7.25.

2. A 35-year-old housewife is brought into casualty in a drowsy state. She is incoherent with slurred speech and her gait is unsteady. She is icteric and has multiple spider naevi on her face and chest.

3. A 67-year-old man with chronic obstructive pulmonary disease is admitted with headache, sore throat, nausea and vomiting. His wife complains of tiredness and lethargy for the last week, ever since they arrived at their holiday caravan.

4. A 21-year-old student is admitted with agitation, paranoid delusions and hallucinations. His temperature and blood pressure are elevated and his pupils are dilated but reactive.

5. A 50-year-old labourer in a farm presents with hypersalivation, excessive sweating, abdominal cramps and diarrhoea. He has hypotension and bradycardia.

Answers to 19.6

1. **J. Salicylates.** The clinical picture of pyrexia, tachypnoea, diaphoresis and metabolic acidosis is suggestive of severe salicylate poisoning. The complex pathophysiology of salicylate toxicity results in stimulation of the CNS (tachypnoea leading to respiratory alkalosis and compensated for by bicarbonate diuresis), uncoupling of oxidative phosphorylation, inhibition of the Krebs cycle dehydrogenase enzymes and amino acid metabolism (leading to metabolic acidosis) and interference with platelet and vascular haemostasis.

2. **E. Ethanol.** This patient with clinical evidence of chronic liver disease, incoherent speech and unsteady gait has had an alcoholic binge. Severe ethanol intoxication may cause stupor, hypothermia, hypoglycaemia and convulsions.

3. **B. Carbon monoxide.** It is likely that there was inadequate ventilation in their caravan when using gas appliances. The man, with a limited respiratory reserve, is affected more than his wife from tissue hypoxia caused by carbon monoxide.

4. **A. Amphetamines.** Amphetamines cause excitability, euphoria, paranoia, dilated pupils (also caused by cocaine, quinine and tricyclics), hypertension and hyperthermia (also caused by theophylline, anticholinergics and monoamine oxidase inhibitors). Convulsions, rhabdomyolysis and cardiac arrhythmias may occur in severe cases.

5. **G. Organophosphates.** This worker in a farm may have been exposed to organophosphorus during crop-spraying or sheep-dipping. They are absorbed through the bronchi, intact skin and the gut and inhibit acetylcholinesterase activity. Onset of symptoms usually occurs rapidly with inhalation and within 12 h of skin contamination. The clinical features are initially due to the muscarinic effects and later due to a combination of nicotinic and muscarinic actions of acetylcholine. Weakness, paralysis, pulmonary oedema with excessive bronchial secretions, hyperglycaemia, convulsions and coma may occur.

ADVERSE DRUG REACTIONS (ADR) AND DRUG INTERACTIONS

19.7 For each of the following scenarios, select the most likely responsible ADR or drug interaction.

A   Carbamazepine ADR
B   Diclofenac/aspirin interaction
C   Gold ADR
D   Lithium ADR
E   Lithium/bendroflumethiazide
F   Methotrexate ADR
G   Penicillamine ADR
H   Propranolol ADR
I   Warfarin ADR
J   Warfarin/trimethoprim interaction

1. A 50-year-old man with uncontrolled psoriasis presents with cough and dyspnoea.

2. A 70-year-old man with hypertension presents with severe bradycardia (pulse rate 35 bpm) 2 days after his treatment was adjusted in his general practitioner's surgery.

3. A 50-year-old patient with a history of bipolar depression was recently found to be hypertensive. He now presents with vomiting, diarrhoea and ataxia.

4. A 75-year-old woman with rheumatoid arthritis attends the hospital regularly for her treatment. She presents to her general practitioner with troublesome diarrhoea and abdominal pain.

5. A 35-year-old woman with a history of multiple pulmonary emboli has also had treatment for her urinary tract infection. She presents to her general practitioner with spontaneous bruising.

Answers to 19.7

1. **F. Methotrexate ADR.** This patient with intractable psoriasis was probably put on methotrexate. Pulmonary toxicity starting with cough and dyspnoea is one of the major adverse reactions associated with this drug.

2. **H. Propranolol ADR.** This is a severe reaction to propranolol, probably because the patient had a co-existing sinoatrial disease. This is easily missed unless there is a history of dizzy spells and the pulse is taken.

3. **E. Lithium/bendroflumethiazide interaction.** This patient is probably on lithium, which has a narrow therapeutic range, with plasma concentration of 0.4–1 mmol/L; a level in excess of 2 mmol/L leads to toxicity. The symptoms include vomiting, diarrhoea, ataxia, weakness, dysarthria and muscle twitching. Thiazide diuretics reduce the urinary excretion and increase the plasma concentration of lithium.

4. **C. Gold ADR.** It would seem that this patient who is under regular follow-up has been started on gold therapy. Diarrhoea with or without abdominal pain is the most common side-effect of oral gold therapy. A bulking agent such as bran might help, but in obstinate cases a temporary reduction in dosage becomes necessary.

5. **J. Warfarin/trimethoprim interaction.** This patient on long-term warfarin was presumably treated with trimethoprim for her urinary infection. Spontaneous bruising is a common side-effect of warfarin, particularly when its anticoagulant effect is enhanced, as in this case, by trimethoprim.

SIDE-EFFECTS OF DRUGS

19.8 In the following scenarios, a disease is described for which a particular drug has been given but unfortunately an adverse reaction has occurred. Select the suspected drug from the list given.

A   Amiodarone
B   Amoxicillin
C   Carbimazole
D   Diazepam
E   Digoxin
F   Haloperidol
G   Lisinopril
H   Lorazepam
I   Nitrofurantoin
J   Quinine

1.   A 45-year-old Welsh patient with schizophrenia has been brought into A&E from a neighbouring psychiatric hospital. The accompanying nurse says that he had been making good progress with the treatment given, but for a day or so he has been unwell with low blood pressure. His pulse rate is 100 bpm, BP 100/60 mmHg and his rectal temperature is 35°C.

2.   A 45-year-old English fitness enthusiast was treated for atrial fibrillation, which was initially difficult to control. Recently, he has found that during his exercises, he gets muscular pains and feels very weak. At times, he feels so fatigued that he has to abandon his exercises.

3.   A 35-year-old housewife of African origin presents with a sore throat. Her full blood count shows a low neutrophil count. She had recently developed hyperthyroidism for which she was receiving some treatment.

4.   A 45-year-old housewife of Mediterranean origin is admitted with acute haemolytic anaemia. She was recently treated for a urinary tract infection.

5.   A 42-year-old Welsh business executive is referred by a marriage guidance counsellor who suspects that he may be suffering from amnesia for recent events. His wife complains that he tells her lies about his whereabouts and deliberately misleads her about where he has been when he is not with her. In the recent past, he has had a very stressful time and is being treated by his doctor for agitated depression.

Answers to 19.8

1. **F. Haloperidol.** Of the many side-effects of the phenothiazine group of drugs, hypotension and interference with temperature regulation are the two often missed. These effects are dose-related and may remain undetected until dangerous hypotension or hypothermia develops in an elderly patient living alone. For this reason, these drugs should be prescribed with caution for patients over 70 years of age.

2. **A. Amiodarone.** As there was some difficulty in controlling this patient's ventricular rate, we can assume that doctors had used amiodarone after having tried digoxin. Side-effects affecting the thyroid (hypo- and hyperthyroidism), muscles (myopathy), nerves (neuropathy), lungs (alveolitis, fibrosis), liver (hepatitis) and the skin (phototoxicity, pigmentation) have all been reported. If the drug is withdrawn early, myopathy is reversible, though it takes a long time to recover.

3. **C. Carbimazole.** This drug can cause sudden bone marrow suppression resulting in agranulocytosis. Before prescribing this drug, the doctor must explain all the possible side-effects to the patient and ask the person to report any symptoms and signs of infection, especially sore throat. The drug should then be stopped immediately.

4. **I. Nitrofurantoin.** This patient of Mediterranean origin probably had glucose-6-phosphate dehydrogenase (G6PD) deficiency. This makes the person susceptible to developing acute haemolytic anaemia if exposed to some drugs such as dapsone, nitrofurantoin, primaquine, quinolones and sulphonamides. G6PD deficiency occurs in most places in Africa, Asia, Southern Europe and Mediterranean regions.

5. **H. Lorazepam.** This patient was probably given lorazepam, which belongs to the benzodiazepine group of drugs, for his agitated depression. Amnesia is known to be one of the side-effects of this group, but it is particularly common and troublesome with lorazepam, which is a very effective anxiolytic agent and is also used as a preoperative sedative.

AVAILABILITY OF DRUGS

19.9 For each of the following drugs, select the correct feature regarding its availability in the UK.

A   Can be sold in any shop
B   Can be sold only by a pharmacist
C   Can be supplied only on an NHS, but not a private, prescription
D   Can be supplied only on prescription (NHS or private)
E   Can be prescribed only by a psychiatrist
F   Can be prescribed only by a registered dentist
G   Can be supplied only on a private prescription
H   Can be supplied only on prescription and in a special pharmacy
I   Can be supplied only on prescription, but attracts no NHS fee
J   Is always illegal to supply

1.   Paracetamol capsules.

2.   GTN spray.

3.   Methadone replacement to a registered drug addict.

4.   Combined oral contraceptive pill.

5.   Cannabis.

Answers to 19.9

1.   **A. Can be sold in any shop.** Paracetamol can be sold in any shop. In an attempt to reduce the severity of overdose in the UK, a limit has recently been placed on the number of tablets that can be sold in a single package.

2.   **B. Can be sold only by a pharmacist.** GTN spray is available without prescription provided it is dispensed by a registered pharmacist. An increasing number of supermarkets are opening pharmacies in their stores but they are allowed to sell such drugs only when a pharmacist is actually on the premises and oversees the sale.

3.   **D. Can be supplied only on prescription (NHS or private).** Methadone is available on prescription and is licensed as an adjunct for the treatment of opiate addicts. It need not be prescribed by a psychiatrist but doctors who regularly supply drug addicts must be registered. Although some drugs are 'black-listed' from the NHS list, a legal drug may be prescribed by a doctor on either an NHS or private prescription. General practitioners are discouraged from providing private prescriptions to their NHS patients.

4.   **I. Can be supplied only on prescription but attracts no NHS charges.** Prescriptions for contraceptives do not incur charges to the patient. When used in high dosage as the 'morning-after pill', combined contraceptives are available without prescription in pharmacies.

5.   **J. Is always illegal to supply.** Cannabis, unlike many other drugs of abuse such as diamorphine and amphetamines, can never be legally prescribed.

TOXICOLOGY

19.10 For each of the following patients admitted to hospital following an overdose, select the most typical clinical feature you might expect to find.

A   Coagulopathy
B   Hyperglycaemia
C   Hyperventilation
D   Metabolic alkalosis
E   Occulogyric crisis
F   Oral burns
G   Respiratory acidosis
H   Skin bullae
I   Tinnitus
J   Ventricular tachycardia

1.   A 62-year-old woman with a long psychiatric history has been using barbiturates to help her sleep at night. She is discovered collapsed in bed with an empty bottle of her tablets on the floor.

2.   A 57-year-old man has struggled to keep his farm in difficult financial circumstances over the last 5 years. He receives a final demand for payment from his bank. Later that day his wife rushes him to hospital after finding that he has tried to swallow weedkiller.

3.   A 27-year-old man visits a general practitioner complaining of a headache. While he is in the doctor's room, he steals some ampoules of drugs that have been left lying in an open bag. Later that night, he injects himself with one of the ampoules that is labelled 'Maxalon'.

4.   A 17-year-old student is taken to hospital by her mother after she admits taking 100 paracetamol tablets the previous afternoon.

5.   A 46-year-old woman is transferred to the acute medical ward after being found in a disturbed state on the psychiatric ward. She has been taking tricyclic antidepressants for several years and has managed to take a large overdose by persuading a visitor to bring in all the tablets she had left at home.

Answers to 19.10

1.   **H. Skin bullae.** Barbiturates are rarely prescribed in modern
     medicine but they were very popular sedatives and narcotics in
     the past. The benzodiazepines are now used in preference
     because they have less addictive and abuse potential (although
     still not negligible). Some patients remain on barbiturates if
     they were prescribed many years ago since they are dependent
     upon them. Skin bullae are a characteristic feature of overdose
     with these agents.

2.   **F. Oral burns.** Paraquat is a component of a number of
     weedkillers and even small amounts are fatal. The oral and
     oesophageal burns are severe and painful but, as the paraquat
     is absorbed, a fatal myocarditis or rapid renal failure results. In
     very small, non-fatal dosage, long-term disability is caused by
     progressive pulmonary fibrosis.

3.   **E. Occulogyric crisis.** Drugs should never be left unattended or
     in a place where others might be tempted to steal them.
     Maxalon™ is a trade name for metoclopramide and, together
     with neuroleptics, may cause an acute dystonic reaction.
     Treatment is with an anticholinergic drug such as procyclidine.

4.   **A. Coagulopathy.** An early feature of paracetamol-induced
     liver failure is coagulopathy due to inability to produce the
     vitamin K dependent coagulation factors in the liver. The
     International Normalized Ratio (INR) is an important prognostic
     indicator in cases of paracetamol overdose.

5.   **J. Ventricular tachycardia.** Serious rhythm disturbances may
     complicate tricyclic overdose. The patient must be monitored
     for 36–48 h since arrhythmias may be delayed.

20

Emergency medicine

EMERGENCY ROOM DECISIONS

20.1 **For each of the following patients, select the most appropriate decision.**

A   Immediate needle decompression
B   Insertion of a chest drain
C   Request aortic arch angiography
D   Request chest X-ray
E   Request D-dimer
F   Request spiral CT pulmonary angiography
G   Request troponin
H   Request urgent echocardiography
I   Request V/Q scan
J   Thrombolysis (if no contraindication)

1. A 30-year-old asthmatic patient becomes suddenly breathless and complains of chest pain. His respiratory rate is 30/min, pulse 120 bpm, oxygen saturation on air 80% and BP 85/60 mmHg. His trachea is deviated to the left and there are absent breath sounds on the right side with hyper-resonance on percussion.

2. A 55-year-old hypertensive patient has a sudden onset of severe central chest pain associated with a tearing sensation in the interscapular area in his back. There is a difference of blood pressure of over 20 mmHg between his two arms. His ECG is normal and his chest X-ray shows a widened mediastinum.

3. A 55-year-old man is admitted to A&E with a 2-h history of severe central chest pain radiating to his left arm. He has been given 'MONA' (morphine, oxygen, nitrate and aspirin). The ECG shows ST elevation in the anterior leads with reciprocal changes in the inferior leads.

4. A 70-year-old female patient with a history of COPD had a hemicolectomy for colonic cancer 10 days previously. She now has pleuritic pain in the left side of her chest, feels breathless and also has coughed up blood on a few occasions. Her ECG shows sinus tachycardia of 110/min and partial right bundle branch block. Her chest X-ray shows chronic scarring in her lungs.

5. A 30-year-old man has symptoms and ECG changes consistent with acute pericarditis. He suddenly deteriorates with a fall in BP, elevated jugular venous pulse and muffled heart sounds.

Answers to 20.1

1. **A. Immediate needle decompression.** This patient has a left-sided tension pneumothorax – *a life-threatening condition requiring immediate needle decompression.* Time should not be wasted on arranging a chest X-ray; an X-ray just confirming a tension pneumothorax without urgent treatment is evidence of negligence!

2. **C. Request aortic arch angiography.** This patient has aortic dissection. Aortic dissection occurs in three groups of patients:
   a. those with connective tissue disease with weakness in the wall of the aorta, e.g. Marfan's syndrome; (b) those with atheromatous aorta; and (c) those with trauma, typically in deceleration injuries.

3. **J. Thrombolysis.** This patient has acute myocardial infarction. Early thrombolysis is indicated to limit myocardial damage.

4. **F. Request spiral CT pulmonary angiography.** This patient has pulmonary embolism. D-dimer is only used as a negative predictor (to rule out) in low probability cases. In patients with chronic lung disease, a V/Q scan may not be sensitive or specific enough for diagnosis.

5. **H. Request urgent echocardiography.** This patient has developed cardiac tamponade. The signs of hypotension, raised jugular venous pulse and muffled heart sounds are called 'Beck's triad'. Bedside urgent echocardiography will confirm the diagnosis and help guide pericardiocentesis.

Medico-legal issues

IMPLICATIONS OF DISEASE

21.1 Each of the following patients seeks advice about the future effect of a current medical condition. Select the most appropriate statement from the list of options.

A   Can never drive a car again
B   Can never drive a school bus again
C   Can never hold a firearms certificate
D   Can never work again
E   Cannot be employed as a healthcare worker
F   Cannot be treated on an intensive care unit
G   Cannot drive a car for at least 1 year
H   Cannot go swimming ever again
I   Cannot work as an orthopaedic surgeon
J   Should never drink alcohol again

1. A 28-year-old school nurse is found to have type 1 diabetes mellitus.

2. A 26-year-old doctor is found to be hepatitis B e-antigen (HBeAg) positive.

3. A 56-year-old physiotherapist has had type 2 diabetes for 10 years and complains of deteriorating vision. On examination, he has diabetic retinopathy that requires laser treatment. In addition, he has widespread changes of retinitis pigmentosa.

4. A 19-year-old student nurse celebrates her birthday by going to a nightclub. She drinks alcohol to excess and also takes half a tablet of what is described as 'ecstasy'. Later that night, while she is asleep, she is witnessed to have a single generalized fit.

5. A 38-year-old hospital administrator with previous convictions for drink-driving is admitted to hospital complaining of abdominal pain. Investigations include a liver biopsy that shows cirrhosis.

Answers to 21.1

1. **B. Can never drive a school bus again.** People taking insulin are able to hold licences to drive ordinary cars (providing they do not have a history of serious hypoglycaemia or significant problems with eye-sight). They are also allowed to apply for firearms certificates. However, they are banned from certain professions (e.g. recruitment to armed forces) and are not allowed to hold the public service vehicle licences required to drive buses, taxis or trains.

2. **I. Cannot work on as an orthopaedic surgeon.** Hepatitis B is a highly infectious disease spread by body fluids. The presence of the e-antigen suggests active viral replication and makes transmission of the disease even more likely. Such an individual would not be allowed to work as a surgeon or in other situations where the infection is likely to be passed on to patients. He could go swimming if he chose, or drink alcohol (although this would be unwise). He would be a risk to others if treated on an intensive care unit but this would not be a reason to deny him treatment. He could be employed as a healthcare worker provided it were in a setting where there was little risk of others being exposed to his body fluids.

3. **A. Can never drive a car again.** The type 2 diabetes is not a particular problem, even if it has led to retinopathy, providing that the eye-sight is well preserved. However, advanced retinitis pigmentosa causes severe restriction of peripheral vision and this will lead to the loss of a driving licence.

4. **G. Cannot drive a car for at least 1 year.** People with epilepsy cannot drive a car for 3 years after their last fit, or 1 year after nocturnal fits. This woman does not have epilepsy as she has had only a single seizure. Nevertheless, a single seizure also precludes driving for 12 months.

5. **J. Should never drink alcohol again.** Alcoholic liver disease is no bar to working in the health service, holding firearms or driving (unless banned from doing so). The cirrhosis is irreversible but the patient should be told never to drink alcohol again since it will hasten the deterioration.

LEGAL IMPLICATIONS IN THE UK

21.2 **Each of the following scenarios requires a particular action that has statutory or legal implications in the UK. Select the most appropriate of these from the list of options.**

A Attracts a fee that is subject to income tax
B Cannot be cremated
C Is always an illegal action
D Must be cremated
E Must be notified to the Public Health Laboratory Service
F Must be referred to the coroner
G Requires the signature of the hospital consultant responsible for the case
H Requires no death certificate
I Requires the consent of relatives
J Requires the signature of the patient's general practitioner

1. A mother who is 20 weeks' pregnant has a miscarriage. There are no signs of life on delivery. She would like to arrange a funeral service followed by a cremation.

2. A 98-year-old man is admitted to hospital complaining of severe abdominal pain and dies 12 h later. The doctor suspects a diagnosis of ischaemic colitis but is not completely sure and would like to arrange a post mortem.

3. A 48-year-old woman is admitted to hospital with meningococcal septicaemia and dies 4 days later. The diagnosis has been confirmed by blood cultures.

4. A patient with rheumatic valvular heart disease and a permanent pacemaker is admitted to hospital with worsening heart failure and dies 9 days later. The relatives would prefer a quiet funeral followed by cremation.

5. A pathologist wishes to collect samples of pancreatic tissue from post mortems so that he can study the accumulation of somatic mutations with age.

Answers to 21.2

1. **H. Requires no death certificate.** A death certificate is required at the death of all individuals that have previously been born with signs of life, whatever the gestational age. However, deliveries prior to 24 weeks' gestation with no signs of life are legally miscarriages and have neither birth nor death certificates. The mother is free to arrange a funeral, burial or cremation without specific legal impediments.

2. **F. Must be referred to the coroner.** Several categories of death must be referred to the coroner. These include any death in which foul play is suspected, death due to occupational disease and within 1 year of an assault. It is often not possible to be completely certain of the cause of death. Although doctors commonly fill out certificates in these situations, when the cause of death is not known, the case should be referred to the coroner. In this scenario, reporting the death to the coroner will ensure a coroner's post mortem that does not require consent from the relatives. Death occurring within 24 h of admission to hospital should at least be discussed with the coroner.

3. **E. Must be notified to the Public Health Laboratory Service.** Several communicable diseases, including meningococcal disease, require notification. In this case, since the patient died, the coroner must also be informed.

4. **A. Attracts a fee that is subject to income tax.** The cause of death seems clear and a death certificate can be filled in. It does not need the signature of either the general practitioner or the hospital consultant. The patient may be cremated but the pacemaker must be removed since there is a risk of explosion otherwise. A fee is payable for both the cremation (but not death) certificate and the removal of the pacemaker. These fees must be declared for income tax purposes.

5. **I. Requires the consent of relatives.** The situation regarding post mortem tissue retained for research purposes has attracted huge publicity recently. Tissue cannot be taken from coroner's post mortems. A hospital post mortem may be undertaken with the consent of relatives and, during the consent procedure, it should be made clear that tissue may be retained for research purposes. Current debate centres on the precise information that must be given to relatives for the consent to be informed and valid (e.g. how much tissue will be retained, for how long and what will be done with it). The issue is complicated by the fact that consent for post mortems is usually taken by a junior medical doctor who may be unaware of the plans of the pathologist.

Index

405